M000022888

THE PCOS Diet COOKBOOK

Easy and Delicious Recipes and Tips for Women with PCOS on the Low GI Diet

Nadir R. Farid M.D., FACP
co-author of The *New Glucose Revolution: Living Well with PCOS*

Norene Gilletz
author of *Healthy Helpings* and *The Low Iodine Diet Cookbook*

YOUR HEALTH PRESS | Second Edition

The PCOS Diet Cookbook: Delicious Recipes and Tips for Women with PCOS on the Low GI Diet
Your Health Press

Second Edition copyright© 2012, Your Health Press.
All recipes copyright© Norene Gilletz, 2007, 2012.
All other text copyright© Your Health Press, 2007, 2012.

Some of the recipes in this book appear in Healthy Helpings, copyright© 2006, by Norene Gilletz, and were adapted with kind permission from Whitecap Books, Vancouver, B.C.

All trademarked products appear herein minus the registered trademark symbol.

All rights reserved. No part of this publication may be reproduced, stored in a retrieval system, or transmitted, in any form or by any means, electronic, mechanical, photocopying, recording, or otherwise, without the permission of the author.

Important Notice
The purpose of this book is to educate. It is sold with the understanding that the author and publisher shall have neither liability nor responsibility for any injury caused or alleged to be caused directly or indirectly by the information contained in this book. While every effort has been made to ensure its accuracy, the book's contents should not be construed as medical advice. Each person's health needs are unique. To obtain recommendations appropriate to your particular situation, please consult a qualified healthcare provider. The low iodine diet is not a diet for the general public, but a specific, temporary diet for thyroid cancer patients.

Design of print and digital editions: Anita Janik-Jones
Cover recipe: Florida Water à la Doris (recipe page 120)
Cover Photo: istockphoto.com

ISBN: 978-0-9851568-6-2

OTHER BOOKS AVAILABLE BY NORENE GILLETZ

The New Food Processor Bible: 30th Anniversary Edition, Whitecap (2011)

The Frequent Fiber Cookbook: Easy and Delicious Recipes and Tips for People on a High Fiber Diet, Your Health Press (2009)

Norene's Healthy Kitchen, Whitecap (2007)

Healthy Helpings, Whitecap (2006)

The Low Iodine Diet Cookbook: Easy and Delicious Recipes and Tips for Thyroid Cancer Patients, Your Health Press (2005)

Second Helpings, Please!, Gourmania, (1968)

MicroWays, Gourmania, (1989)

OTHER BOOKS BY NADIR R. FARID

The New Glucose Revolution: Living Well with PCOS by J. Brand Miller, N.R. Farid and K. Marsh. Avon, New York (2004)

The New Glucose Revolution: Managing PCOS by J. Brand Miller, N.R. Farid and K. Marsh. Hodder Headline, Australia (2004)

Academic Books Edited by Dr. Nadir R. Farid

The Molecular Basis of Thyroid Cancer, Kluwer Academic Publishers, Boston (2004)

Immunogenetics of Autoimmune Disease, CRC Press Inc., Boca Raton, FL (1990)

Molecular Aspects of Autoimmunity, N.R. Farid and C.A. Bona, eds., Academic Press, Orlando, FL (1990)

Immunogenetic Aspects of Endocrine Disorders, N. R. Farid and Allan R. Liss eds., New York (1988)

Anti-Idiotype Molecular Mimicry, N.R. Farid and S. Linthicum, eds., Springer-Verlag, New York (1988)

HLA in Endocrine and Metabolic Disorders, Academic Press, New York (1981)

ACKNOWLEDGMENTS

This book is dedicated to the late Nadir R. Farid, M.D., a pioneer in using low glycemic diets to treat PCOS.

We are indebted to the meticulous work of our Low GI Diet Nutritional Advisor on this project, Elana Hirschowitz, B. Pharm., BSc. Diet (SRD.

TABLE OF CONTENTS

PART 2: COOKING AND RECIPES

Chapter 4: Breakfasts ... 43

Cereals
Cheeses
Eggs
Fruit Dishes
Breads
Spreads
Muffins
Cakes for Breakfast

Chapter 5: Lunches ... 81

Soups
Salads and Dressings
Sandwiches, Fillings and Spreads
Fish Dishes
Chicken and Turkey
Pasta
Vegetable Dishes

Chapter 6: Dinners ... 181

Soups
Salads and Dressings
Side Dishes
Fish Dishes
Chicken and Turkey
Beef
Pasta
Marinades and Sauces
Vegetarian Entrées

WHAT IS PCOS?

PCOS stands for polycystic ovarian syndrome, which now affects a staggering number of women. One-quarter to one-third of women of reproductive age suffer from PCOS. The vast majority of women with PCOS also have severe insulin resistance. Although insulin resistance is at the root of PCOS, it can occur outside of it as well. We now know that a full 50 percent of the population is insulin resistant, a condition in which the body "resists" the normal functions of the hormone insulin.

Insulin resistance and PCOS are a major health hazard for women of all ages. PCOS, in particular, is a risk factor for diabetes, heart disease, fatty liver, uterine cancer, serious sleep disorders, depression, multiple miscarriages, multiple pregnancies and preeclampsia.

Fortunately, PCOS is manageable. A program that includes medications that sensitize the body to insulin, as well as lifestyle changes that address the signs and symptoms of PCOS, can be remarkably effective. One of the key elements of this program is following a low glycemic index diet, also known as the *low GI diet*.

LOW GI EATING

Low GI eating emphasizes foods containing carbohydrates that break down slowly, and thus release sugar into the bloodstream slowly, keeping the blood sugar more stable. These foods are called *low glycemic index* or *low GI* foods. The glycemic index (see the Appendix) ranks foods with a value of 0 to 100 according to their effect on blood sugar levels. Changes in blood sugar produced by a given food are measured against the rise in blood sugar produced by a load of sugar, or sucrose, which is 100 percent. To qualify as low GI, foods should have an index of 60 percent or less; those above 60 percent are considered high GI.

HOW FOOD AFFECTS INSULIN

One of the important influences of a low GI diet is its effect on the body's capacity to secrete insulin. A high GI diet results in large peaks of insulin secretion by the pancreas, whereas low GI eating results in a steady secretion of insulin. This means that on a high GI diet you might experience "sugar crashes" where you find that after a meal you get tired or sleepy, and then a few hours later become very hungry, resulting in the need to eat more to keep your blood sugar stable.

Insulin is the principal hormone involved in the laying down (or accumulation) of fat in the body. This is because one of insulin's functions is to inhibit the release of fat from fat stores. Since fat stores around the midriff (meaning "belly fat") are especially sensitive to the effects of insulin, too much insulin makes using abdominal fat as a source of fuel exceedingly difficult. When fat gradually accumulates around the midsection of girls or women, it's a typical sign of PCOS, but more generally it's a sign of insulin resistance in *both* women and men.

America's obesity epidemic over the last three decades has coincided with an overall increased intake of carbohydrate-containing foods, many of which are high GI. What's made matters worse is our tendency to eat one or two large meals a day. This results in tsunami-size insulin peaks, which predispose us to weight gain, as well as a host of symptoms and side effects that are a result of excess insulin in the blood. To address these symptoms and side effects, low GI eating also calls for frequent healthy low GI snacks to maintain steady low levels of insulin in the blood.

If you happen to have PCOS, low GI eating will help to reduce your symptoms and halt the progression of your disease. Low GI eating will also decrease insulin levels, making it easier for your body to burn fat.

There are other advantages to a low GI diet. It can:
- Lower your blood fats (or triglycerides)
- Allow you to feel fully satisfied after eating
- Reduce your risk of developing diabetes and other diseases

- Improve your physique (since you'll be losing weight, and helping your body to redistribute its fat stores, you'll also lose "belly" fat)
- Allow for better quality sleep
- Improve your overall sense of well-being

SIGNS AND SYMPTOMS OF PCOS

The signs of PCOS range from the subtle, such as excess facial hair (clinically known as hirsutism), to what's called the "full house" syndrome. The latter can mean no periods, obesity, excessive body hair, diabetes and cardiovascular disease. It's apparent from this rainbow of symptoms that PCOS is not just an ovarian disease. PCOS affects the whole body. The underlying cause of PCOS is excess insulin in the blood, which occurs as a result of insulin resistance.

PCOS can start any time during a woman's reproductive life. Since insulin resistance rises naturally just before puberty, PCOS can even be seen in girls as young as 10 or 12 years. In fact, we now know that girls who experience early puberty (or the appearance of pubic hair and breasts at age seven or eight) have a very high risk of subsequent PCOS.

The early diagnosis and treatment of girls and women is vital. Only through early diagnosis and treatment can we avoid seeing PCOS progress to its more severe, "full house" syndrome. If you suspect you have PCOS, speak to your doctor about testing (discussed further on in this chapter). PCOS *is* manageable. Management is rooted in lifestyle changes (such as exercise, adopting a low GI diet and practicing stress-reduction techniques) as well as medications that address the problem of insulin resistance.

WHAT TO LOOK FOR

- Early puberty, or the appearance of pubic hair and breasts at age seven or eight
- Delayed or absent puberty
- Irregular periods, or no periods at all
- Acne, particularly if it first appears in adulthood
- Excess body hair or facial hair (also called hirsutism)

7

- Unexplained fatigue
- Sugar craving
- Hypoglycemia, or low blood sugar, occurring after or between meals
- Excess weight around the waistline
- Infertility
- Mood swings
- Hot flashes (characterized by heat intolerance and excess sweating) in young women
- Sleep disorders, particularly sleep apnea (meaning that you might stop breathing in your sleep)
- Recurrent miscarriages
- Milk leaking from the breasts (or inappropriate lactation)
- Low blood pressure noticeable when you stand up suddenly, or after exercise
- Rough, dark skin in the neck folds and armpits, known as "Acanthosis nigricans"

Some of these signs and symptoms, such as fatigue, are a product of insulin resistance, whereas others can be linked to the excess production of male hormones from the ovaries and adrenal glands. Consult your doctor if you notice several of the signs and symptoms on this list. You don't have to have all or even most of the signs or symptoms of PCOS; even a handful of them may indicate that PCOS (or another disease) is present.

A PCOS diagnosis is made via blood tests and ultrasound. Since not all patients satisfy the diagnostic criteria for the disease, early diagnosis requires a high index of suspicion, which is subsequently confirmed by testing. This means that doctors have to suspect PCOS is present before they diagnose it.

What the diagnostic tests look for are high levels of serum testosterone, low levels of the sex hormone-binding globulin (which is the protein that ferries testosterone and estrogens around the body) and high levels of lutenizing hormone (LH) compared to follicle stimulating hormone (FSH). On ultrasound examination, bulky ovaries with 10 or more peripheral cysts are also an indicator of PCOS.

CAUSES OF PCOS

Like many common disorders such as Type 2 diabetes and heart disease, PCOS is known as a *complex common trait*, implying that environmental as well as genetic factors contribute to its development. Environmental factors can include a high GI diet (containing foods that rate high on the glycemic index), little or no exercise and stress.

Recent studies have actually shown that stress causes insulin resistance. Fat deposits in the body differ according to location, and those in the midsection and inside the tummy are particularly sensitive to insulin. Insulin induces an enzyme that converts steroid precursors to cortisol; hence the common appearance of persons who are insulin-resistant and those on steroids

The Role That Genes Play in PCOS

Some ethnic groups such as Hispanics, Polynesians and East Indians experience higher rates of both insulin resistance and PCOS. Even in the general population, PCOS tends to run in families. In fact, some research has shown that the PCOS "trait" as seen in female family members may also show up in male members of the same family. Men experience this trait differently, however, usually displaying high serum dehyroepiandosterone, weak adrenal androgen, high rates of frontal baldness, and central obesity. Not infrequently, a woman with PCOS will also have a family history of diabetes, high blood pressure or high cholesterol.

Research shows that the genes implicated in PCOS are involved in insulin action and in the production of sex hormones. It's actually the relationship between insulin resistance, ovarian hormones and increased pituitary stimulation of the ovaries that accounts for all the signs and hormonal features of PCOS. Interestingly, research has also shown that stress can induce changes in the body that lead to insulin resistance. And, stress accelerates the genetic changes associated with aging, also known to be a factor in PCOS.

The Role That Insulin Plays in PCOS

Insulin resistance is a common condition in which the body has to secrete more than average amounts of insulin. This is because a resistance to insulin has developed. Insulin is a hormone essential for life, but in excess it can cause many undesirable signs and symptoms, including PCOS.

A simple blood test, which measures your fasting glucose along with insulin, can help diagnose insulin resistance. However, some research suggests that half of all patients with PCOS actually have a normal fasting glucose/insulin relationship, despite the fact that they were proven to be insulin resistant by more technically demanding investigations. Even lean women with PCOS can be insulin resistant, although with weight gain insulin resistance gets worse. Insulin resistance results in the excess production of hormones from the ovaries and adrenal glands, which accounts for the symptoms of PCOS. Excess insulin has a tendency to lay fats cells around the waist and inside the tummy, as well as to cause fat infiltration of the muscles, liver and even heart. Because continued excess insulin gradually compromises the ability of the pancreas to secrete insulin, to the extent that the pancreas simply cannot cope, it's no surprise that insulin resistance is the most important risk factor for the development of diabetes.

Insulin does its job by latching on to a specific insulin receptor, whose concentration decreases (thus weakening the signal insulin transmits to the cell). However, ovarian insulin receptors do not weaken, and thus the ovary is the target of persistent insulin action. Insulin both directly and indirectly stimulates the growth of the ovarian tissue between the eggs, which actually comprises the bulk of the ovary. This part of the ovary makes sex hormones, and the enzymes involved in this synthesis are also turned on by insulin.

Estrogen is made in the ovary through the conversion of testosterone. In PCOS this conversion process is frequently flawed, resulting in excess testosterone. Excess testosterone causes male-patterned body changes in women. These changes can include male-patterned excess facial and body hair (called hirsutism), abdominal weight gain and, in the case of some women, the development of male muscular features.

Excess insulin and testosterone also make the area at the base of the brain, known as the hypothalamus, more sensitive. As a result, the signal it sends to the pituitary gland becomes more frequent and more intense. The pulses of luteinizing hormone (LH) that the pituitary secretes periodically become larger and more frequent, causing further ovarian stimulation and creating a vicious cycle of ovarian stimulation and sex hormone over-secretion. To make matters worse, insulin is responsible for the conversation of weak male and female sex hormones to more potent forms, which "reside" in the body's fat stores. This complex and chaotic interplay between endocrine glands accounts for all of the symptoms of PCOS, which are further magnified by eating a high GI diet, not exercising, and stress.

WHY PCOS CAN PUT YOU AT RISK

PCOS is a risk factor for many serious medical conditions, which is why it's important to minimize symptoms as early as possible. PCOS can increase your risk of developing the following:

- Metabolic syndrome, also known as "Syndrome X" (see further)
- Type 2 diabetes
- Autoimmune thyroid diseases, such as Hashimoto's disease (resulting in hypothyroidism or an underactive thyroid) or Graves' disease (resulting in hyperthyroidism, or an overactive thyroid)
- Coronary artery disease
- Stroke
- Early miscarriage (in the first trimester)
- Multiple pregnancies (being pregnant with twins or more)
- High blood pressure
- Preeclampsia (a condition in pregnancy)
- Depression
- Uterine cancer
- Alzheimer's disease

It's important to remember that this list represents a worst-case scenario, and conditions such as uterine cancer very rarely develop, even in untreated cases of PCOS.

Metabolic Syndrome

One of the consequences of severe, progressive insulin resistance is metabolic syndrome, which is truly the last "way station" an insulin resistant person reaches before going on to develop diabetes. Its origins and the cellular mechanisms it involves have fascinated scientists over the last few years. Thus there is much scientific work now being done on insulin resistance and metabolic syndrome, sometimes with unexpected results.

One practical development concerns how doctors estimate a person's risk for developing metabolic syndrome and its consequences, such as heart disease. Rather than using Body Mass Index (BMI) testing, a hip/waist ratio of weight distribution is examined. In metabolic syndrome, the higher the ratio, the greater the risk. Interestingly, there is evidence that fat stored in the buttocks area instead of the abdominal area may offer protection from obesity-related diseases such as metabolic syndrome, or Type 2 diabetes.

Not infrequently severe PCOS is associated with metabolic syndrome. I have, therefore, suggested that PCOS ought to be considered one of the "signs" of metabolic syndrome. Overweight women with PCOS frequently have at least two to three additional characteristics of metabolic syndrome, such as:
- A high hip/waist ratio, also known as central obesity
- High blood sugar (in the fasting state, before breakfast or after meals)
- High blood triglycerides, or "trigs"
- High levels of small, dense cholesterol particles
- Low levels of HDL or "good" cholesterol
- Fatty liver, also known as non-alcoholic steatohepatitis, or NASH

Clearly the list of characteristics associated with metabolic syndrome can only be assessed through laboratory or radiology testing. It's important to discuss these options with your doctor. Left untreated, metabolic syndrome can lead to more serious conditions.

MANAGING PCOS

PCOS needs to be identified and treated early so that it doesn't progress. As discussed, PCOS can predispose you to serious health problems, including central obesity, hirsutism, fatty liver and diabetes. But to manage PCOS successfully you'll have to be prepared to make certain lifestyle changes. You'll also have to stick with these changes to maintain good health and control your PCOS. And although drugs are regularly used to sensitize the body to insulin, drugs alone have limited benefit unless they're accompanied by the following:

- Low GI eating (the focus of this book!)
- Exercise
- Stress reduction techniques

These lifestyle changes will help to enhance your sense of well-being, as well as your self-esteem. For more information on hair removal and hirsutism, visit- *www.yourhealthpress.com*.

SUCCESS STORIES

It's difficult to explain how life changing it can be to obtain a definitive diagnosis of PCOS, and be able to finally take charge of your health. I have selected five cases from my own patient population to illustrate what I call the "success stories." These are patients who suffered with a collection of odd symptoms until PCOS was finally recognized. Three of the cases will be shared here; two of the cases will be shared in Chapter 1. I have changed the names of these patients to protect their confidentiality.

Case History 1

"Nancy" was 32 years old and was referred to me because of a lump on her thyroid. I did a fine needle biopsy of the lump, and found it was benign. After taking a careful history, I learned Nancy had symptoms of severe fatigue, steady weight gain (despite being careful), acne before her periods, unpredictable periods, and extreme mood swings—which were *not* due to any thyroid problem. Through blood tests, I found she was insulin resistant. I started her on a low GI diet and regular exercise, and prescribed metformin, an insulin-sensitizing drug, to make her body more sensitive to its own insulin.

When she first presented to me, she weighed 165 pounds, and was quite frumpy in appearance and dress. Within three years, she dropped down to 130 pounds, developed a curvy figure (instead of a fat midsection) and reported boundless energy. She also reported a promotion at work, which I attribute to greater self-esteem. The accurate diagnosis of PCOS, combined with lifestyle changes and an insulin-sensitizing drug, transformed this woman's entire physique.

Case History 2

"Elizabeth" was a successful investigative journalist struggling with infertility; she wrote many health stories and had interviewed me once. She was 36, and her husband was 41. The interval between her periods had been getting later and later, and her husband apparently had a low sperm count. This couple began fertility treatments and went through a cycle of IVF. During that cycle, Elizabeth was informed that the quality of her eggs was poor, and could not be harvested. She came to see me because of various things I had spoken about in our interview, which included signs of PCOS. I reviewed her medical history, did a full workup, and discovered that she was insulin resistant, with signs of mild PCOS.

I started her on metformin and a low GI diet, as well as a regular exercise routine. This quite petite woman weighed about 120 pounds, but once she began her regimen, soon lost about 7 pounds, which made a big difference to her physique. She did a second IVF cycle, and was told that the quality of her eggs was high. They were actually able to harvest many of these eggs, which were easily fertilized. Elizabeth had a successful pregnancy and gave birth to twins. Again, an accurate diagnosis transformed struggles with infertility, and deep anxiety over it, into a beautiful life.

Case History 3

"Joan" was an obese 15 year-old, weighing about 250 pounds. She had large buttocks, but reported to me that at puberty her weight ballooned, regardless of how carefully she ate. She also reported extreme fatigue, sleep problems and hot flashes, as well as dark, rough skin on her neck and underarms.

Her periods were very irregular, and her GP suspected she had PCOS and referred her to me. I put her on the PCOS management program: the low GI diet, regular exercise and metformin. Five months after starting this program, she weighed in at about 185 pounds, and reported much more energy and better sleeping. Since then she has continued to lose weight, but the most significant improvement has been in her self-esteem and sense of well-being. Had this 15 year-old girl remained undiagnosed, terrible consequences would have ensued with her self-esteem and socialization. Again, an accurate diagnosis prevented this fate.

THE LOW GLYCEMIC INDEX CUPBOARD: WHAT TO BUY AND HOW TO SHOP FOR THE LOW GI DIET

If you've read the Introduction, you'll see that there are many specific choices for the low glycemic index (GI) diet. This chapter will help you shop for the food products you'll need to properly follow this diet. You'll also learn how to interpret the nutrition labels on your packaged foods to determine whether they're actually low GI foods.

To make this chapter easy to understand, I want you to imagine you're in a supermarket, and ready to do a large shopping trip. Get your cart. Now, let's walk through the aisles together, starting with the inside aisles, where we usually find the packaged food items, and finishing with the outside aisles, where we normally buy our meats, produce, baked goods, and so on.

PACKAGED FOOD IN THE INSIDE AISLES: WHAT'S OKAY, WHAT'S NOT

The glycemic index runs from 0 to 100 and usually uses glucose—which has a GI value of 100—as the reference. The effect other foods have on blood sugar levels are then compared with this. In simple terms, the GI index tells us whether a food raises blood sugar levels dramatically, moderately or just a little bit. Foods that have only a slow, small effect on blood sugar have a low GI value, while those causing a rapid and massive rise in blood sugar have a high GI value. There are many books and websites that list the GI index for different foods, and we provide some tables of commonly used foods, which you'll need for most of the recipes in this book. (See the Appendix.) The GI covers only carbohydrates, such as fruits and juices, potatoes, rice, pasta, breads, cereals, etc., which contain sugars, starches and different types of fiber.

Food values may vary slightly depending on the source, but in general they should be roughly the same. Many lists divide the foods into categories of low, medium/moderate and high. Foods in the low category usually have a GI value of 55 or less (see Page 292); in the medium/moderate category, a GI value of 56 to 69 (see page 293); and in the high category, a GI of 70 or more (see page 294).

You might be surprised by some of the foods included in the low and high categories. Rice cakes and Bran flakes actually have a high GI value, even though you may have learned that these foods are great weight-loss choices. Meanwhile, salted peanuts and milk chocolate have a low GI value, but they're still very high in calories. Many of the foods that have a low GI value but are high in fat should be limited as well. *Remember: foods only appear on the GI index if they contain carbohydrate.* This explains why you won't find foods like fresh meat, chicken, fish, eggs and cheese in GI lists, even though they have dense calories. But they are low GI! To further complicate matters, you may find certain processed foods, like sausages or chicken nuggets, on some GI lists because they contain flour! Some foods cause glucose levels to rise quickly after you eat them. The result is a virtual "gush" of glucose into the bloodstream, which in turn results in a rating of these foods as high GI. Other carbohydrate foods cause glucose levels to rise more slowly—more like a "trickle"—and this results in a rating of these foods as low GI.

JUDGING A GI VALUE BY ITS PACKAGE

How can you tell what the GI value of a packaged food item, which contains many different ingredients, will be? First, the overall nutrient content of a food will affect its GI. For example, fat and protein affect the absorption of carbohydrate. This helps to explain why chocolate, which is high in fat, has a low GI value.

How you cook a food and the degree of processing it has undergone also affect its GI. So does, for example, the ripeness and variety of a fruit. Even the structure of the carbohydrate itself influences the GI. For example, processed instant oatmeal has a higher GI than traditional rolled oats. This is because, as a result of the processing, the starch in instant oats is more easily exposed to digestive enzymes, causing it to break down and enter the bloodstream more rapidly. Meanwhile, some foods have low GI values because they're packed with fiber. Fiber acts as a physical barrier, slowing down the absorption of carbohydrate into the blood.

EYEBALLING GLUCOSE

There are several kinds of sugars in the foods we eat; some are natural, and some processed. Natural sugars include fructose (fruit sugar), lactose (milk sugar), and maltose (grain sugar). These natural sugars have lower GI values, and will not cause a spike in blood sugar levels to the extent that sucrose (or ordinary table sugar) will. So, in packaged food items, what you especially need to watch for are foods *high in sucrose* or foods that come with the phrase "added sugar" on their packaging; these are sugars that manufacturers add to foods during processing.

Foods containing fruit juice concentrates, invert sugar, regular corn syrup, honey or molasses, hydrolyzed lactose syrup or high-fructose corn syrup (made out of highly concentrated fructose through the hydrolysis of starch) all have added sugars. And many people don't realize that pure, *unsweetened* fruit juice is still a potent source of sugar, even when it contains no added sugar. Extra lactose, dextrose and maltose are also contained in many of our foods. In other words, these products may have naturally occurring sugars anyway, and then *more* sugar is thrown in to enhance consistency, taste and so on. The best way to know how much sugar is in a product is to look at the nutritional label. If sugars aren't mentioned on the label, look at "total carbohydrates."

However, *how fast* that sugar ultimately breaks down and enters your bloodstream greatly depends on the amount of fiber in your food, how much protein you've eaten and how much fat accompanies the sugar in your meal. This is what helps determine the overall GI rating of a meal.

Why Are Sugars Added?

Sugars are added to foods because they can change their consistency and, in some instances, act as a preservative, as in jams and jellies. Sugars can increase the boiling point or reduce the freezing point in foods; sugars can add bulk and density, and make baked goods do wonderful things, including help yeast to ferment. Sugars can also add moisture to dry foods, making them "crisp," or balance acidic tastes found in foods like tomato sauce or salad dressing. Invert sugar is used to prevent sucrose from crystallizing in candy; corn syrup is used for this purpose as well.

Since the 1950s, a popular natural sugar in North America has been fructose, which has replaced the sucrose in many food products in the form of high-fructose syrup (HFS), made from corn. HFS was developed in response to high sucrose prices and is very cheap to make. In other parts of the world, the equivalent of high-fructose syrup is made from whatever starches are local, such as rice, tapioca, wheat or cassava. According to the International Food Information Council in Washington, D.C., the average North American consumes about 37 grams of fructose daily.

"Sugar-Free"

Sugar-free in the language of labels simply means "sucrose-free." However, this doesn't mean the product is carbohydrate-free, as in dextrose-free, lactose-free, glucose-free or fructose-free. Check the labels for all ingredients ending in "ose" to find out the sugar content; you're not just looking for sucrose. Watch out for "no added sugar," "without added sugar" or "no sugar added." This simply means: *we didn't put the sugar in, God did*. Again, reading the number of carbohydrates on the nutrition information label is the most accurate way to find out the amount of sugar in the product. Fruits and vegetables are discussed at the end of this chapter.

SWEETENERS

What does a low GI dieter do when she's craving sweets? Products with certain sweeteners are an option, but only if in liquid or tablet form. Sweeteners in granulated forms (e.g., Splenda) should not be used at all, since these substitutes contain Maltodextrin as a bulking agent. Maltodextrin is very high GI product, and is to be avoided in all areas. In fact, from a GI rating standpoint, a small amount of sugar may even be a better choice.

Most artificial sweeteners will be classified as low GI because they don't affect your blood sugar levels since they don't contain sugar. But they may contain a few calories. It depends on whether a given sweetener is classified as nutritive or non-nutritive.

Nutritive sweeteners have calories or contain natural sugar. White or brown table sugar, molasses, honey and syrup are all considered nutritive sweeteners. *Sugar alcohols* (see below) are also nutritive sweeteners because they're made from fruits or produced commercially from dextrose. Sorbitol, mannitol, xylitol and maltitol are all sugar alcohols. Like ordinary sugar, sugar alcohols contain only four calories per gram, and will affect your blood sugar levels like ordinary sugar. How *much* sugar alcohols affect your blood sugar levels depends on how much is consumed, and the degree of absorption from your digestive tract.

Non-nutritive sweeteners are sugar substitutes or artificial sweeteners; they don't have any calories and will not affect your blood sugar levels. Examples of non-nutritive sweeteners are saccharin, cyclamate, aspartame, sucralose and acesulfame potassium.

Acceptable Daily Intake for Sweeteners

Note: Only liquid or dissolved tablet sweeteners should be used; powdered forms are not acceptable for the low GI diet.

Sweetener	Intake based on mg/kg body weight
Aspartame	40
Ace-K	15
Cyclamate	11
Saccharin	5
Sucralose	15 (US) / 9 (Canada)

Source: Canadian Diabetes Association, "Guidelines for the Nutritional Management of Diabetes Mellitus in the New Millennium. A Position Statement." Reprinted from Canadian Journal Diabetes Care 23 (3): 56–69.

Xylitol, also called wood sugar or birch sugar, is a five-carbon sugar alcohol that's used as a sugar substitute. It can be extracted from birch, raspberries, plums and corn and is primarily produced in China. Xylitol, gram for gram, is roughly as sweet as sucrose, but contains 40 percent less food energy.

FOODS IN JARS AND TINS

There are many canned and jarred foods available to the low GI dieter. Here are things to have on hand and pick up when strolling the aisles:

- Tuna (preferably in water)
- Salmon (preferably in water)
- Sardines (preferably in water)
- Tomatoes and tomato paste
- Corn
- Fruits (not packed in syrup)
- New white potatoes
- Vegetables (asparagus, carrots, green beans, mushrooms, etc.). Marinated vegetables packed in jars are great as snacks and side dishes. An added benefit is the vinegar they contain, which helps lower the GI of the foods you eat along with them. Examples include sun-dried tomatoes, artichoke hearts and olives.
- Dried fruits and nuts, especially walnuts and nut bars
- Capers
- Marinated vegetables
- Roasted peppers
- Pickles

THE OUTSIDE AISLES

What you need to eat on the low GI diet is usually found in the outside aisles of any supermarket or grocery store. Outside aisles stock the foods you can buy at outdoor markets: fruits, vegetables, meat, eggs, fish, breads and dairy products. Natural fiber is also found in the outside aisles. But remember: foods you buy in the outside aisles can be high in fat unless you select wisely. Fat content may also affect the GI values. Whole milk, for example, has a low GI value because it's packed with protein and fat.

HOW INGREDIENTS AFFECT THE GI VALUE OF A MEAL

The outside aisles will help you select low GI ingredients wisely. But how you cook a food, the degree of processing and the ripeness and variety of a fruit, for example, can also affect its GI value. Yellowish green bananas are a good example. They have a lower GI value than the darker yellow, spotty bananas. Processed instant oatmeal has a higher GI value than traditional rolled oats because the starch in instant oats is more easily exposed. This is why any baking recipes in this book that call for oatmeal will specify rolled oats. If you use instant oatmeal rather than rolled oats, the recipe will still turn out, but your food will have a higher GI value.

Meanwhile, some foods have low GI values because they're packed with fiber (discussed further on), which acts as a physical barrier, slowing down the absorption of carbohydrate into the blood. It's important to remember that GI charts only identify the effect different foods have on bloods sugar levels when they're eaten on their own. Once you put them together in a meal, the mixture of foods will completely change the GI value of what you're eating. As a guideline, the more low GI foods you include in a meal, the lower the overall GI value of that meal. All the recipes in this book take into account a balance of ingredients. Together these ingredients produce a low to medium GI-value meal, which is also nutritionally balanced.

Food Acidity

The more acidity there is in food, the more slowly it's emptied from the stomach—and the more slowly it's digested and turned into blood sugar. Foods that are acidic, such as oranges and sourdough breads, have low GIs. Adding acid to a meal in the form of vinegar (found in many salad dressings) or lemon juice can therefore help lower the GI value of that meal. Adding roughly four teaspoons of vinegar in the form of vinaigrette dressing at an average meal can actually lower blood sugar by 30 percent. Recipes with acidic foods can also balance higher GI ingredients. So just to recap, adding pickles and other acidic vegetables to meals can lower the GI values of those meals. Adding lemon juice or vinegar to recipes has the same effect—the GI values of those meals are lowered.

The Importance of Fiber

A key component in lower GI foods is fiber. Complex carbohydrates are foods that are high in fiber. Fiber is the part of a plant your body can't digest. It comes in the form of both water-soluble fiber (which dissolves in water) and water-insoluble fiber (which doesn't dissolve in water but instead absorbs water). Soluble fibers, such as those found in apples, rolled oats and beans and other legumes, tend to slow digestion, resulting in a low GI. Including kidney beans or chickpeas in a salad or adding an apple as the dessert to a meal will lower that meal's overall GI—thus producing a slower and more subtle rise in after-meal blood sugar levels.

Soluble fiber also lowers the "bad" cholesterol, or LDL, in your body. Experts aren't entirely sure how soluble fiber works its magic, but one popular theory is that it gets mixed into the bile the liver secretes, and forms a type of gel that traps the building blocks of cholesterol, thus lowering your LDL levels. It's akin to a spider web trapping smaller insects. Sources of soluble fiber include oats or oat bran, legumes (dried beans and peas), some seeds, carrots, oranges, bananas and other fruits. Soybeans are also high sources of soluble fiber. Soluble fiber helps delay the absorption of glucose into your bloodstream, which not only improves blood sugar control but helps to control post-meal peaks in blood sugar.

Insoluble fiber doesn't affect your cholesterol levels at all, but it does regulate your bowel movements. As insoluble fiber moves through your digestive tract, it absorbs water like a sponge and helps form your waste into a solid matter faster, making the stools larger, softer and easier to pass. Without insoluble fiber, your solid waste just gets pushed down to the colon or lower intestine as usual, where it's stored and dried out until you're ready to have a bowel movement. High-starch foods are associated with drier stools. Ignoring "the urge" only makes the situation worse, as the colon will continue to dehydrate the waste. This makes it harder and difficult to pass, a condition known as constipation. Insoluble fiber will help to regulate your bowel movements by speeding things along. It's also linked to lower rates of colorectal cancer. Good sources of insoluble fiber are wheat bran and whole grains, skins from various fruits and vegetables, seeds, leafy greens and cruciferous vegetables (cauliflower, broccoli or Brussels sprouts).

For more information about fiber, see *The Frequent Fiber Cookbook*, which can be a nice companion to the book you're reading right now.

Finding High-Fiber, Low GI Grains and Bread

Rethinking "bread" is critical for people on a low GI diet. Even breads made with whole-grain flour can still be high GI. Flour actually has to be 100 percent stone-ground whole wheat—or another soluble fiber product (such as oats, oat-bran, wheat germ, or All Bran) needs to be used—for a bread to be low GI. This book contains only bread recipes that produce low GI bread. For a bread to be low GI, it needs to be labeled as whole grain, multigrain or 100 percent stone ground. Rye bread can also be low GI, but must be labeled as being whole meal or sourdough rye. Other types of "acceptable" breads include those made with soya, sunflower seeds or linseeds.

Although whole-grain breads are good sources of insoluble fiber (flax bread is particularly good because flax seeds are a source of soluble fiber, too), they may not be low GI unless they're 100 percent whole grain. The problem lies in understanding what's actually "whole grain." For example, there's an assumption that because bread is dark or brown, it's more nutritious; this isn't so. In fact, many brown breads are simply enriched white breads dyed with molasses. ("Enriched" means that nutrients lost during processing have been replaced.) Whole-wheat pita breads are considered classic low GI breads. A good rule is to simply look for the phrase "whole wheat," which means that the wheat is, indeed, whole.

Cereals

A list of low GI cereals appears on page 295. In general, choose rolled oats over quick-cooking or instant oatmeal. Shredded Wheat, All Bran, or higher fiber cereals are lower in GI than Bran Flakes, Corn Flakes, and so forth.

Baking Ingredients

If you're planning to bake, and the recipe uses whole-wheat flour or plain white flour, be aware that these both have high GI values. (The insoluble fiber added to whole-wheat flour does not bring the GI down). *The flour needs to be 100 percent stone ground.* It *is* acceptable to have plain flour provided that there's a soluble fiber component to the recipe. Recipes using flour labeled as all-purpose flour, flour, bread flour, whole-wheat flour, etc., are all high GI flours. However, if enough soluble fiber is in the recipe to counteract the high GI effect of the flour used, the recipe is acceptable. Examples would be ingredients such as rolled oats, a number of apples, applesauce, wheat germ, raw carrots, protein foods such as yogurt or buttermilk, and other acidic ingredients. We were careful to assess each recipe in this book on this basis, in order to produce something that's tasty *and* low GI.

Many baking recipes contain cornstarch, which is a high GI thickening agent. Yet when there are relatively small amounts of cornstarch in a recipe that contains a lot of protein, the GI will still be kept relatively low, and only these kinds of recipes containing cornstarch are included in this book. But as a general rule, be aware that low GI thickening agents are flour or oat bran.

Breadcrumbs, while a common ingredient in many recipes, have been omitted from this cookbook because it's difficult to find packaged breadcrumbs that are whole grain unless you make them yourself; if you want to add breadcrumbs to any of these recipes, be sure to use whole-grain or low GI breadcrumbs. Again, as far as baking is concerned, powdered sugar substitutes or sweeteners should not be used as they contain substantial amounts of maltodextrin, a high GI bulking agent. These sweeteners have a higher GI than sugar itself. However, liquid sweeteners usually do not contain maltodextrin; nor do tablet sweeteners. Tablet sweeteners need only be dissolved in a very small quantity of water and added to the recipe. If bulk is required for the recipe, it's preferable to use sugar or fructose rather than powdered sugar substitutes or sweeteners.

Fats and Oils

It's important to focus on the right fats and oils for your cooking needs. You generally want to opt for an oil that's monounsaturated—in other words, a "good fat."

Here's a good list of oils to buy for the low GI diet, oils which are also *good for you*:

- Olive oil is always a great choice because it's 74 percent monounsaturated, which means it can actually lower cholesterol levels and protect against heart disease. Olive oil looks even better when compared to saturated and trans-fats, which stimulate cholesterol production in the body, causing the arteries to be blocked. And you can use olive oil for just about everything; Mediterranean cultures even sprinkle it on bread in place of butter, and over pasta (with a little garlic) in place of fattier cream or tomato sauces. So, when dressing salads, olive oil is actually a far better bet than some of the "non-fat" options available today. As for baking, it used to be that olive oils were considered too strong for baking. These days, however, there are many light olive oils on the market that boast a very neutral taste. So there's rarely, if ever, any need to stray from this "protective" cooking tool. In our baking recipes here, we still recommend canola oil (see next).
- Other monounsaturated oils are canola, flax seed, peanut, soybean, and avocado. Canola is second in line to olive oil, and is 50 percent monounsaturated. Canola oil is extracted from rapeseed, which comes from the cabbage family of plants.
- Non-stick (and non-fat) cooking sprays are also fabulous for use in low-fat cooking because they completely eliminate the need for butter. These sprays also come in flavors like lemon and garlic, which add a whole lot of taste without the fat. If you coat your saucepan with cooking spray first, you'll only need to add a very small amount of oil for low-fat stir-fries and so on. In most cases, just a teaspoon is enough—especially with the flavored varieties, which pack a wallop of taste.

Pastas and Rice

Whole-wheat pastas are lower in carbs, and brown rice is lower in carbs than white pasta or white rice. There are now a variety of low GI pastas and rice to choose from. As long as pasta is made of Durum wheat and is cooked "al dente" (see below) it's low GI. A good medium GI choice of rice is Basmati, brown or long grain rice. As a general rule, avoid any quick-cooking or instant starches.

Many of the pasta sauces in this cookbook will go beautifully with any of the whole-wheat or high-fiber pastas. For even lower carb options, spaghetti squash, steamed spinach, broccoli or other cooked vegetables can substitute for pastas, rice or other carbs normally required for sauces. As a general rule, cooked foods have higher GIs than uncooked foods. One of the reasons is because cooking causes starches to swell, which makes them easier to digest and they therefore convert into glucose more quickly. The amount of cooking time can affect the GI, too. When pasta is cooked only until it's al dente (firm), it has a low GI; when pasta is overcooked and becomes soft and mushy, it has a higher GI.

Beverages

The general advice is to stick with two to five liters of water per day. Caffeine is to be kept to a minimum (no more than two cups per day). Sodas, including diet sodas, are not recommended as they contain phosphates that leach calcium from the bones. Alcohol is also not recommended as it's full of empty calories and tends to turn the appetite on; people find they lose weight faster and feel better if they stop drinking altogether once they begin low GI eating.

Meats and Fish

All fresh meats are fine. Lean meats are preferable, as are fish and seafood. Fish and seafood are actually very highly recommended components of the low GI diet. But when it comes to meat, choose from:

- Chicken, Cornish hen, and turkey (all without skins). You can also substitute ground turkey for ground beef in burgers.
- Lean beef (round, sirloin, chuck, loin). Look for "choice" or "select"

grades instead of "prime," and lean or extra-lean ground beef (with no
more than 10 percent fat).
- Lean veal, ham, and pork (tenderloin, loin chop) and lean lamb (leg, arm, loin).
- Red meats, but only once or twice per week; pork and lamb are particularly fattening.
- Chicken breast or drumstick instead of chicken wing or thigh.
- Exotic meats, such as emu, buffalo, rabbit, pheasant, and venison. These have less total fat than animals commonly raised for market.

Bulk Food Items

Bulk food items are generally more affordable than the processed or packaged variety you may be used to eating. They're also high-fiber items, and when properly stored, they last forever! When preparing for a low GI diet, here are some suggestions:
- Dried beans and peas (great for soups and stews).
- Rolled oat flakes over packaged or "instant" cereal.
- Barley for use in soups (as well as on its own). Also high in fiber.
- Basmati rice, brown or wild rice and whole grain pastas. In general, it's always a good idea to opt for those grains that have undergone the least amount of processing.
- Whole grains such as bulgar and couscous as another alternative to breads or a common white starch. Both of these grains, when added to vegetables, can transform a healthy starch into a hearty meal!
- Natural peanut butter, as long as it comes without any added sugars.

Fruits and Vegetables

The lowest GI fruits to choose from include all varieties of citrus fruits (e.g., grapefruits and oranges) as well as apples, apricots, cherries, mulberries, peaches, pears, plums, strawberries and kiwi. Dried fruits such as apple slivers, apricots and sultanas are low GI, but raisins are not. And as for vegetables, most leafy green and cruciferous vegetables are low GI, including beans (with the exception of Haricot beans or refried beans), lentils and chickpeas. It's best not to opt for sweet corn and peas, as both have a higher GI value. There are certain root vegetables, such as parsnips, which are also high GI. Carrots, on the other hand, have a low to medium GI value.

What's worth considering too, especially in our discussion of fruits and vegetables, is a relatively new concept called the glycemic load (GL). Although the glycemic load assesses the impact of carbohydrate consumption by taking the glycemic index into account, it also goes a step further. While a given GI value represents the speed at which a particular carbohydrate turns into sugar, it doesn't represent the *quantity* of carbohydrate you'll find in a serving of that particular food. Let's put it this way: the carbohydrate in a melon has a high GI value. But there's actually very little of it, which means that the melon's glycemic load is relatively low. A GL of 20 or more is considered high; a GL of 11 to 19, medium; and a GL of 10 or less, low. Foods that have a low GL almost always have a low GI. So even if a melon is moderate to high in GI, a *slice* of melon has a totally acceptable GL value. Thus a slice, now and then, is just fine.

MORE SUCCESS STORIES
Case History 4

"Sally" was a patient that who lived in Belgium, whose sister suggested she come see me about her struggle with infertility. Sally got pregnant after two years struggling to conceive, and then had seven first-trimester miscarriages. However, her Belgian obstetrician could find no reason for these miscarriages. I did a full workup on Sally and found that she had normal fasting blood glucose tests and insulin levels, but since we now know that 50 percent of patients with PCOS *will* have normal fasting blood glucose tests, I thought I'd start her on the program of low GI eating, exercise, metformin and stress management.

In six weeks, Sally lost 11 pounds, had improved energy and slept better. She got pregnant again eight weeks later, and this time had a successful pregnancy.

It turns out the repeated miscarriages were due to a hormonal decrease in LH during the "luteal" phase of her pregnancy as a result of mild PCOS, and it was easily corrected with the addition of progesterone in her first trimester.

Case History 5

"Frances" is a patient we use on our website as an example of "before and after." At 4 feet 10 inches, Frances weighed more than 165 pounds. She was a "text-book" case of PCOS, and suffered from severe fatigue and hot flashes. I began Frances on the PCOS program of a low GI diet, exercise and metformin.

Four years later, Frances weighs 119 pounds. She reports feeling a profound sense of well-being, and consistent high energy. She also reports significant changes in her marriage, and it's easy to see that this as a testimony to her vastly improved self-esteem. Again, an accurate diagnosis of PCOS made a world of difference for Frances.

CHAPTER TWO

LOW GI MEAL PLANNING: A SAMPLE LOW GI MENU

The three-day menu that follows illustrates what an ideal low GI diet looks like in real life. All of the recipes listed in this chapter can be found on the corresponding page numbers; recipes can also be mixed and matched to suit your taste buds.

DAY ONE
Breakfast

Old-fashioned oatmeal made from rolled oats with skim milk and peaches
100% stone-ground whole-wheat toast with no-sugar-added marmalade jam

Mid-Morning Snack

Apple dipped in all natural peanut butter (with no sugar added)

Lunch

Lighter Chopped Egg Salad (see page 124) on 100%
stone-ground whole-wheat bread
Cup of mixed berries and/or slice of melon

Mid-Afternoon Snack

Healthier Hummus (see page 278) with celery or carrot sticks

Dinner

Green Split Pea and Barley Soup (see page 85)
Grilled Moroccan Salmon (see page 216)
Green Salad with Balsamic Salad Splash (see page 93)

Dessert (optional)

Orange Creamy Dream (see page 255)

Beverages

Any beverage is fine so long as it does not have sugar or added sugar. For example, unsweetened coffee or tea, or either beverage sweetened with liquid or tablet sweeteners is fine. Water or other beverages with liquid or tablet sweeteners, such as Xylitol (available in specialty stores), are also fine. Unsweetened juices in moderation are fine, but do stick to two glasses per day.

DAY TWO
Breakfast

Shredded Wheat with skim milk
Fruit Smoothie (see page 51)

Mid-Morning Snack

Assorted nuts and/or seeds with unsweetened apple juice

Lunch

Best Cottage Cheese (see page 46) on 100%
stone-ground whole-wheat bread
Green Salad with Orange Balsamic Vinaigrette (see page 106)
One firm, yellow banana

Mid-Afternoon Snack

Sweet Potato Chips (see page 273)

Dinner

New-Wave Gazpacho (see page 86)
Chicken with Bulgur and Mushrooms (see page 225)
Minted Peas with Red Peppers (see page 200)

Dessert (optional)
Hot Chocolate (see page 25)

DAY THREE
Breakfast
Two eggs any style with 100% stone-ground whole-wheat toast
Better than Butter Spread (see page 63)
Sliced apple and yogurt

Mid-Morning Snack
Slice of Jumbleberry Crisp (see page 53) with a glass of skim milk
One orange

Lunch
The Best Chicken Soup (see page 90)
Oriental Cucumber Salad (see page 107)

Mid-Afternoon Snack
Spinach and Herb Dip (see page 281) with celery sticks and carrot sticks

Dinner
Greek-Style Lentil Soup (see page 84)
Sweet and Sour BBQ Brisket (see page 237)
Beans and Carrots Amandine (see page 188)

Dessert (optional)
Chocolate Chip Bran-ana Muffins (see page 250)

CHAPTER THREE

LOW GI ON THE TOWN

This chapter is designed to address the question: *What should I do when I have to eat out?* In a world of life-threatening food allergies and dozens of special health diets, restaurant cooks and wait staff have been trained to accommodate us, and most, if not all, will adjust.

Although you can never know for sure what's in your food unless you're cooking it yourself, there has to be some level of trust in a good restaurant with a responsible manager and chef. Unlike other diets, one misstep on occasion is not going to cause ill health for the GI diner. This chapter will help you avoid pitfalls while dining out so you can stay as low GI diet-friendly as possible. Today, with so many "low carb" options, eating out has never been easier.

THE FIRST STEPS

The hospitality industry isn't called the hospitality industry for nothing, and these days dealing with food restrictions is just one component of good service. Consider taking your first steps in a favorite neighborhood or restaurant district. Most establishments post menus outside, and a quick glance at the night's offerings will often confirm whether or not you'll find something that's low GI-friendly. Once you become familiar with the ingredients that are off-limits to the low GI diner, you'll get to know where these ingredients crop up in various cuisines. You'll then be able to tell at a glance which items on a menu can be altered to suit your needs, and which you'll want to avoid altogether. This way, choosing a restaurant won't be the challenge you feared. And if friends or colleagues have chosen the restaurant for you, consider calling in advance (ideally during off hours) to get a sense of the menu.

STARTERS

Simpler, fresher choices are best, as they're often much easier to dissect. Choose a salad and request, if you can't confirm that the dressing is low GI-friendly, a bottle each of olive oil and balsamic vinegar with some salt and pepper. Some restaurants (particularly Italian) will bring these condiments to your table alongside the dinner rolls or bread, and almost all restaurants will have them on hand in the kitchen.

Soups are fine, so long as they're not made purely from ingredients high in sugars, such as tomato soups or cream of potato. Sticking to chicken-based soups, vegetable-based broths, or legume-based soups is best.

Grilled veggies (or some variation thereof) are a popular item on many of today's menus. They're typically made with olive oil, not butter, and so are a great choice for the low GI diner.

MAINS

Entrées tend to combine food groups, which means it will be more important than ever to *ask questions*. Once you've eliminated the more obvious choices (such as potatoes, white rice and pasta) you can turn your attention to some possible pitfalls. Sauces can be tricky, as they're often prepared in advance with added sugars and "white stuff" such as refined flour. Stuffed dishes (such as stuffed chicken) are typically pre-stuffed with breadcrumbs, which might not be the best option.

If the entrée you want comes with potatoes or rice, take a look at the other available mains. Why not substitute those potatoes for extra salad or veggies or even pasta? Most kitchens, particularly busy kitchens, prefer substitutions to out-and-out requests for a personal chef.

DESSERTS

Obviously, steer clear of commercially prepared baked goods (i.e., anything made at outside bakeries or cake shops), as their ingredients are much higher in sugars and processed flours. Fruit-based pies are usually extremely high in sugar. Sticking to fresh fruit plates, sorbets or even poached fruits is best. Dark chocolate flourless desserts are also better options.

LOW GI AROUND THE WORLD

Thanks to today's global village, eating out is a multicultural experience. Once reserved for the urbanites among us, ethnic diversity is now as close as the nearest town or strip mall—where you'd be hard pressed not to find at least one Chinese restaurant. But how much you have to choose from will naturally depend on your neighborhood, so it's best to familiarize yourself in advance with the challenges of a multicultural menu.

Chinese and Vietnamese Restaurants

Your biggest challenge with these common Asian options is avoiding the sweet sauces that accompany many of the meat and vegetable dishes, as well as high starch items such as noodles and rice—especially the rice! Lower GI alternatives include egg, rice or mung bean noodles. Hoisin sauce, oyster sauce, soy or other dark Asian sauces are very high GI items. In general it's a good idea to:

- Ask if sauces can be served on the side.
- Avoid *lo mein* noodle dishes, as they won't be made with high-fiber pasta. Avoid rice.
- Order dishes that are made on the spot with fresh ingredients, such as a vegetable stir-fry or meat dish. Garlic and herbs are okay.

Greek Restaurants

The biggest culprits here are what come with the meals: lots of rice and potatoes and bread. Otherwise, Greek cuisine offers mostly low GI fare, including delicious souvlaki dinners and whole-wheat pitas. There are also many tasty vegetable options. When in Greek town:

- Ask if you can replace the rice and potatoes that come with most meals with vegetables or salad.
- Consider a Greek salad with feta, but have the dressing (often high in sugar) on the side.
- Remember that fried calamari is often breaded, and thus should be avoided.

- Know that tzatziki (the white dressing or dip that's served as a side with much of Greek fare) is made with yogurt and is high in lactose, but in moderate amounts is fine.
- Make sure (by checking with your server) that any other pre-made offerings have no added sugars.

Indian Restaurants

Indian food is wonderfully varied, but much of it's served in the form of stews or curries. The "bread" that's perfect for the low GI diner at Indian restaurants is the flat, cracker-like *papadum*, which is actually made from lentils. However, many Indian foods are heavily sauced, and are difficult to "diagnose" in terms of ingredients. Most servers at Indian restaurants are used to educating their customers about the ingredients that go into the various dishes, so asking about how the sauces are made is a perfectly good way to go. Sauce-less choices are obviously ideal, and include the delicious (baked) *tandoori* chicken. Additionally:

- Avoid the bread called *naan* and substitute with *papadum*.
- Be aware that Indian cuisine commonly utilizes yogurt for its cooling properties, which can be high in lactose. However, moderate amounts are fine. (And as a general rule, low-fat yogurt is also fine.)
- Avoid gulping down a *lassi*, India's favorite yogurt drink, as it's very sweet and full of sugar.
- Make sure your food is not cooked in *ghee*, which is a butter sauce.

Japanese Restaurants

If you find yourself in a Japanese restaurant, nothing is off-limits except the rice. Stick to rice-less fare, such as *sashimi*, various meat dishes, and so forth. *Tempura* is made with a batter, which could also be a poor choice. However, when balanced with vegetables, *tempura* is fine. Try to limit the teriyaki or soy sauces. Otherwise, enjoy!

Italian Restaurants

The low GI diner can do very well with Italian cuisine and is best selecting durum wheat pastas cooked al dente. This is slightly undercooked pasta, which lowers the starch content of the pasta, and gives you a lower GI value. Thin pastas can also be options in moderation. Some Italian restaurants now offer whole-wheat or high-fiber pastas, which are also fine. But Italian restaurants offer many grilled options as well, and antipasto plates in which cheese figures prominently. Be aware, however, that there are some sneaky pitfalls in traditional Italian fare. They are:

- Breadcrumbs. Many Italian recipes ask for breadcrumbs, so be diligent with your server about this.
- Risotto. Risotto is rice, and not an option for you if you want to avoid starchy foods.
- Bread. Watch the bread before the meal!

Latin Restaurants

These are nice places to be if you want to maintain a low GI diet. Dishes containing guacamole or refried beans are fine. Salsas and tortilla chips are the real culprits, and tortillas (the popular Mexican flatbreads made with corn or wheat) should also be avoided.

Spanish and Cuban restaurants often feature a "tapas" menu. This is a real treat for anyone with food restrictions, as it tends to mean lots of choice (the portions are tiny) and few surprises.

Thai Restaurants

Thai food is sweet and savory, simple and complex. Much of it is low GI-friendly, but much of it is not! What you need to avoid are rice- or rice noodle-based dishes. Cold rice paper used for fresh spring rolls is filled with crunchy fresh vegetables, coriander and rice noodles, and the dipping sauce is on the side. The paper rolls are usually thin enough that in moderation, they should be fine.

Traditional *Pad Thai* is a poor option, since it's mostly noodle based. Coconut dishes can be very sweet, so should be avoided. Stick to broths and meat dishes and you'll be fine.

Other things to watch out for include:

- Fish Sauce. This is used extensively in Thai cooking, so you'll need to ask whether it's high in sugars; if it is, it can come on the side.
- Dipping Sauces. These accompany many of the appetizers. Ask your server how each has been prepared, so you can select wisely.

Fast Food

Fast food is infamous for its hidden sugars, even in food items you wouldn't suspect have such ingredients. Try to drive through all fast food outlets, as there's absolutely no guarantee you'll find low GI-friendly foods other than a salad with no dressing and bottled water. And you don't need a drive-thru for that.

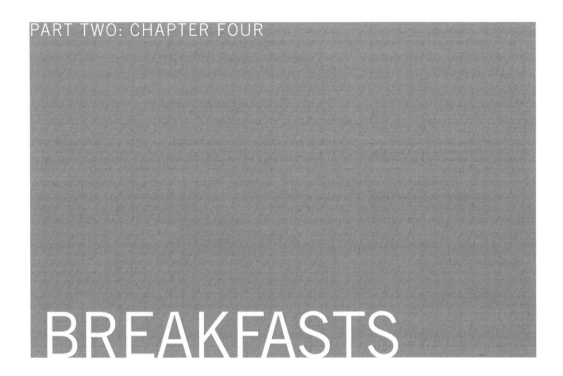

BREAKFASTS

WHAT'S INSIDE

■ CEREALS

Note: *the following cold cereals are all low GI, and are recommended with skim milk and a low GI sweetener (see chapter 1, page 20):*
- *All Bran with Fiber*
- *Bran Buds*
- *Fiber One*
- *Muesli (may depend on the sugar content)*
- *Oat Bran cereals*

Great Granola

Easier to make and healthier than commercial brands, this also makes a great snack. Omitting raisins from the recipe will lower the GI value even more.

    ¼ cup oil
    ¾ cup honey
    ¼ cup maple syrup
    3 cups rolled oats
    ½ cup shredded coconut, optional
    2 tbsp wheat germ, optional
    ½ cup sesame seeds
    ¾ cup chopped, unsalted nuts (pecans, filberts, walnuts, or almonds)
    1 tsp cinnamon*
    1 tsp vanilla
    ½ cup raisins

1. Preheat oven to 350ºF.
2. Combine oil, honey and maple syrup in a large bowl. Add remaining ingredients, except raisins, and mix well. Spread mixture on a large rimmed baking sheet. Bake uncovered for 30 to 35 minutes, or until toasted, stirring occasionally.

3. Stir in raisins. Let cool, stirring with a fork occasionally to break up mixture. Store in an airtight container in a cool, dry place.

Yield: About 6 cups. Can also be frozen.**

Mom's Old Fashioned Oatmeal

> 3 cups hot water
> ½ tsp salt
> 1 ⅓ cup rolled oats

1. Combine hot water, salt and oatmeal in a 3-quart microsafe casserole. Microwave uncovered on HIGH for 8 to 9 minutes, stirring at half time. Stir and let stand for 3 minutes.

Yield: 4 servings. Reheats well.**

Variation:
Top cooked rolled oats with a layer of fresh or frozen blueberries or strawberries, as well as a layer of non-fat yogurt. Sprinkle with cinnamon.

Oat Bran Cereal

1. For 1 serving, measure ¼ cup oat bran cereal into a microsafe bowl (about 20 oz capacity). Add ¾ cup tap water. Microwave uncovered on HIGH for 1 minute, then on MEDIUM-LOW/DEFROST (30%) for 2 minutes.**

**No nutitional analysis available.

■ CHEESES

A piece of your favorite cheese with a slice of low GI toast is ideal at breakfast time. Top with sliced cucumbers to eat cold. Or cover with thinly sliced tomatoes and some salt and pepper, then pop into the toaster oven or under the broiler. Low-fat cheeses are the best choices, and are found in abundance at your grocery store or supermarket. Here are some more ideas:

Best Cottage Cheese (Homemade!)
My cousin Wendy Harrison of England taught me how to make this. It's simply delicious!

1. In a large pot, heat 2 liters (quarts) of milk until simmering (use 1% or skim). Sprinkle in lemon juice (about 4 to 6 tablespoons) until mixture begins to separate into curds and whey. Remove from heat.
2. Pour warm liquid into a cheesecloth-lined colander. Tie ends of cheesecloth and let drain for several hours. (Hang it over the faucet of the sink; put a bowl underneath to catch the whey.) For a firmer cheese, squeeze out most of the liquid. Wrap well and refrigerate.

Yield: About 2 cups. This keeps at least a week in the refrigerator.

41 calories per ¼ cup, 0.6 g fat (0.4 g saturated), 2 mg cholesterol, 7 g protein, 2 g carbohydrate, 7 mg sodium, 48 mg potassium, trace iron, 0 g fiber, 34 mg calcium.

Buttermilk Cheese (Tvarog)
Marina Tagger of Winnipeg, Canada shared this guilt-free, creamy cottage cheese, which is an old Russian recipe.

1. Place 2 liters (quarts) of buttermilk in a large, covered ovenproof casserole. Place in a preheated 375°F oven for 15 to 20 minutes.

It will separate into curds and whey. Drain as directed in Step 2 (see previous page). Calci-yummy!**

Note: *Use the whey that drains off to replace buttermilk when baking low GI muffins, cakes and quickbreads.*

Cheese Pancakes

This recipe is also a Passover dish, and requires matzo meal (found in the Jewish or ethnic foods section at the supermarket). The protein in this recipe counteracts the matzo meal to make this a low GI pancake—almost unheard of!

 1 cup dry cottage cheese (non-fat or low-fat)
 2 eggs plus 2 egg whites
 2 tbsp sugar
 2 tsp melted tub margarine
 ¼ cup non-fat yogurt
 ½ cup matzo meal
 ⅛ tsp salt
 ¼ tsp ground cinnamon*

1. In the processor, process all ingredients until smooth and blended, about 30 seconds. Spray a large non-stick skillet with non-stick spray. Heat on medium heat. Spoon the batter by rounded spoonfuls onto the hot pan. Brown on medium heat on both sides until golden. Serve with yogurt and berries.

Yield: About 12 pancakes.

50 calories per serving, 1.6 g fat (0.4 g saturated), 37 mg cholesterol, 5 g protein, 4 g carbohydrate, 123 mg sodium, 50 mg potassium, trace iron, trace fiber, 26 mg calcium.

**No nutitional analysis available.

■ EGGS

Two eggs any style are perfectly fine for a low GI diet and make the ideal breakfast with a slice of low GI toast (see chapter 1 and also under Homemade Breads). Try your toast with one of the low GI spreads, too (see further). But since cholesterol is a problem for many of you on the low GI diet, here are recipes for yolk-free egg dishes.

Egg Whites, Any Style

> 4–6 egg whites
> salt and pepper, to taste

1. Prepare the egg whites as you would normally: fried or scrambled, with the exception of sunny-side-up or over-easy! Serve plain or with a low GI bread you may have made or purchased. **

Hard-Cooked Egg Whites
How egg-citing, hard-boiled eggs! Use these in a sandwich filling, homemade potato salad or anywhere you use hard-boiled eggs. Two egg whites are the equivalent of 1 egg.

1. Mix 2 egg whites lightly in a 10-oz glass custard cup or small microsafe bowl. Cover tightly with microsafe plastic wrap. Do not vent.
2. Microwave on MEDIUM (50%) for 1 to 1 ½ minutes, depending on how powerful your microwave oven is. Let stand covered for 1 to 2 minutes, until completely set.

Yield: 1 serving. Do not freeze.**

**No nutitional analysis available.

Savory Egg White Omelet

4–6 egg whites
salt and pepper, to taste

1. Combine egg whites with seasonings and mix lightly to blend. Prepare in a frying pan, using a heart-healthy oil or margarine (see chapter 1). Add any of the following ingredients for the most popular egg/omelet mixtures: chopped asparagus, broccoli, red or green peppers, onions, mushrooms, sliced or diced cooked chicken, zucchini, spinach, tomatoes, Italian herbs.**

Sweet Egg White Omelet

4–6 egg whites
cinnamon* to taste

1. Combine egg whites. Prepare in frying pan using non-stick cooking spray, canola or neutral-flavored vegetable oil. Serve plain, or add any of the following low GI fruits to the omelet center: apples, apricots, cherries, peaches, pears, plums or strawberries.

   Sprinkle with cinnamon just before serving.**

■ FRUIT DISHES

Apple and Apricot Pudding (a.k.a. Kugel)

"Out of this world!" according to Joy Bucknoff, who shared her yummy recipe with me. Apple and Apricot Pudding can be served for breakfast, lunch or as a side dish with dinner. This recipe with its dried apricots, lemon juice, eggs and apples counteracts the high GI effect of the matzo meal used.

**No nutitional analysis available.

49

6 eggs, beaten (or 4 eggs plus 4 whites)
½ cup sugar
6 apples, peeled and grated
½ cup matzo meal (available in the Jewish or ethnic foods sections
of your supermarket)
juice of 1 lemon (3 tbsp)
1 cup dried apricots, cut up
2 tbsp sugar mixed with ½ tsp cinnamon*

1. Preheat oven to 350°F. In a large mixing bowl, combine eggs with sugar;
    mix well. Add apples, matzo meal and lemon juice. Mix until smooth.
    Soak apricots in hot water for 5 minutes; drain well. Spray a 7 x 11-inch
    Pyrex casserole with non-stick spray. Spread half of mixture in pan.
    Arrange apricots in a single layer over batter. Top with remaining batter;
    spread evenly. Sprinkle with cinnamon-sugar. Bake at 350°F about
    1 hour, until golden.

Yield: 10 servings. Reheats well. Can be frozen.

*190 calories per serving, 3.6 g fat (1 g saturated), 127 mg cholesterol, 5 g protein,
37 g carbohydrate, 40 mg sodium, 308 mg potassium, 1 mg iron, 4 g fiber, 28 mg
calcium.*

Citrus or Melon Baskets

- *Basket without Handle:* Trim top and bottom of citrus fruit or melon to
  form a stable base at both ends. Cut in half with a V-shaped knife (or
  make uniform zigzag cuts with a sharp knife), cutting all the way through
  to the center. Adjust the last cut to meet the first cut. Separate the halves.
  Use a melon baller to hollow out melon. Pulp from citrus fruit can be
  removed with a sharp paring knife or grapefruit knife. Fill grapefruit,
  orange or melon baskets with colorful fresh fruit salad.

- *Basket with Handle:* Trim bottom of fruit to form a stable base. Cut away 2 wedges from the top side so you're left with a handle in the middle of the basket. Make uniform zigzag cuts around basket and handle with a V-shaped or sharp knife, adjusting the last cut to meet the first cut. (Don't cut through the handle!) Cut away pulp under the handle with a sharp knife. Remove pulp, leaving a shell that is firm enough to hold the filling. Use a small ice cream scoop for watermelon, a melon baller for smaller melons and a grapefruit knife for citrus fruit. A few hours in advance, fill as desired. Trim the handle with overlapping citrus slices anchored with toothpicks. Top each toothpick with a grape or strawberry. Refrigerate until serving time.

Note: Remember to consume melons in moderation!

Fruit Smoothies
Lush slush!

> ½ cup skim milk or yogurt
> ½ cup sliced fruit (e.g., strawberries, peaches)
> ¼ tsp vanilla extract
> 2–3 ice cubes
> sugar or low GI sweetener to taste (1 to 2 tsp sugar or the equivalent in low GI artificial sweetener—see chapter 1, page 21)

1. In a blender or processor, blend the first 4 ingredients together until smooth. Add sweetener to taste. Makes about one cup.

87 calories per serving (with sugar), 0.5 g fat (0.2 g saturated), 2 mg cholesterol, 5 g protein, 16 g carbohydrate, 64 mg sodium, 343 mg potassium, trace iron, 2 g fiber, 163 mg calcium.

With low GI artificial sweetener, one serving has 74 calories and 13 g carbohydrate.

Variations:

- ***Banana Smoothie:*** *Combine ½ banana, ½ cup skim milk, ½ teaspoon vanilla and 1 teaspoon sugar. Blend until smooth. Makes 1 serving containing about 100 calories.*
- ***Banana Yogurt Smoothie:*** *Combine 1 ripe banana, ¾ cup non-fat yogurt or buttermilk, ⅓ cup skim milk, 1 teaspoon honey (to taste) and 3 or 4 ice cubes. Blend until smooth. For a thicker smoothie, use a frozen banana and omit ice. Makes 2 servings.*
- ***Banana Strawberry Smoothie:*** *Combine 1 ripe banana, ½ cup sliced strawberries, ¾ cup orange or pineapple juice (or skim milk), 1 to 2 teaspoons honey and 3 or 4 ice cubes. Blend until smooth. Omit ice cubes if using frozen banana or strawberries. Makes 2 servings.*

Homemade Applesauce

Applesauce makes a wonderful accompaniment to lots of dishes in this cookbook. My grandmother always added a ripe pear, and her applesauce was the best!

8 medium apples
1 Bartlett pear, optional
¼ cup water or apple juice
3–4 tbsp sugar
1 tsp cinnamon*

1. Peel and core the apples and pear. Cut them into chunks. Combine all ingredients (except low GI sweetener, if using—see chapter 1) in a large saucepan. Bring to a boil, reduce heat to simmer and cook partially covered for 20 to 25 minutes, until tender. (To microwave, cook covered on HIGH power for 6 to 8 minutes, or until tender. Stir once or twice during cooking.) Break up applesauce with a spoon, or serve it chunky.

Yield: 6 servings. Freezes well.

124 calories per serving, 0.8 g fat (0.1 g saturated), 0 mg cholesterol, <1 g protein, 32 g carbohydrate, 2 mg sodium, 166 mg potassium, trace iron, 5 g fiber, 14 mg calcium.

Notes:

- *If you have a food mill, cook apples without peeling; wash well before cooking and discard stems. After cooking, put mixture through a food mill. Applesauce will be rosy pink.*
- *If using apple juice, use minimum amount of sugar or low GI sweetener. If you want apples to keep their shape, add sugar after cooking, not before. If using sweetener, add after cooking.*

Variations:

- **Applesauce with Mixed Fruits Compote:** *Use your favorite combination of fruits (e.g., apples, pears, blueberries, strawberries, rhubarb, peaches, plums, nectarines) for a delicious dessert.*
- **Rella's Blueberry Apple Sauce:** *Add 2 cups of blueberries 5 minutes before end of cooking time.*

Jumbleberry Crisp

This is one of those "desserts for breakfast" dishes. My cousin Nancy Gordon of Toronto gave me the idea for this fast and fabulous crisp based on her yummy Bumbleberry Pie. I combined various berries, eliminated the crust, and this delectable dessert is the result. If you're missing one kind of berry, just use more of another. If using frozen berries, don't bother defrosting them. If you don't have apples, add extra berries!

Filling:

1½ cups strawberries, hulled and sliced
2 cups blueberries
1½ cups cranberries and/or raspberries
2 large apples, peeled, cored and sliced

⅓ cup flour (whole-wheat or all-purpose)
⅓ cup sugar (white or brown)
1 tsp cinnamon*

Topping:
⅓ cup brown sugar, packed
½ cup flour (whole-wheat or all-purpose)
¾ cup rolled oats
1 tsp cinnamon*
¼ cup canola oil

1. Combine filling ingredients; mix well. Spray a 10-inch glass pie plate or ceramic quiche dish lightly with non-stick spray. Spread filling ingredients evenly in dish.
2. Combine topping ingredients (can be done quickly in the processor). Carefully spread topping over filling and press down slightly. Either bake at 375°F for 35 to 45 minutes until golden, or microwave uncovered on HIGH for 12 to 14 minutes, turning dish at half time. Serve hot or at room temperature. Delicious topped with a small scoop of low-fat frozen yogurt!

Yield: 10 servings. Freezes well.

202 calories per serving, 6.3 g fat (0.5 g saturated), 0 mg cholesterol, 3 g protein, 36 g carbohydrate, 6 mg sodium, 186 mg potassium, 1 mg iron, 4 g fiber, 25 mg calcium.

Notes:
  • *Topping can be prepared ahead and frozen. No need to thaw before using.*
  • *Prepare crisp as directed, but use 6 to 7 cups of assorted frozen berries and omit apples. Assemble in an aluminum pie plate, wrap well and freeze unbaked. When you need a quick dessert, unwrap the frozen crisp and bake it*

without defrosting at 375°F about 45 minutes.
- *If you're making this dessert in the microwave, place a large microsafe plate or a sheet of waxed paper under the cooking dish to catch any spills!*

Variations:

- *Skinny Version: Reduce oil to 2 tablespoons and add 2 tablespoons water or apple juice to the topping mixture. One serving will contain 178 calories and 3.6 g fat (0.3 g saturated).*
- *Skinniest Version: Substitute 3 tablespoons "lite" margarine instead of ¼ cup oil in the topping mixture. One serving will contain 168 calories and 2.6 g fat (0.4 g saturated).*
- **Fruit Crisp:** *Substitute 6 to 7 cups of assorted sliced fresh (or frozen) fruits and/or berries (peaches, pears, nectarines, blackberries, etc.).*

Peachy Crumb Crisp

Filling:

6 cups peeled, sliced peaches (or a combination of peaches, nectarines and plums)
1 tbsp lemon juice
¼ cup brown sugar, packed
¼ cup flour (whole-wheat or all-purpose)
1 tsp cinnamon*

Topping:

¼ cup brown sugar, packed
½ cup flour (whole-wheat or all-purpose)
¾ cup rolled oats
1 tsp cinnamon*
2 tbsp tub margarine or canola oil
2 tbsp orange juice

1. Combine filling ingredients and place in a sprayed 10-inch ceramic quiche dish. Combine topping ingredients and mix until crumbly. Sprinkle over fruit. Bake at 400°F for 45 minutes. If necessary, cover loosely with foil to prevent over-browning.

Yield: 10 servings. Freezes well.

162 calories per serving, 2.9 g fat (0.5 g saturated), 0 mg cholesterol, 3 g protein, 33 g carbohydrate, 24 mg sodium, 308 mg potassium, 1 mg iron, 4 g fiber, 27 mg calcium.

Variations:
- **Blueberry Peach Crisp:** *Use 4 cups sliced peaches and 2 cups blueberries in the filling. Add 1 tsp grated orange zest.*
- **Blueberry Nectarine Crisp:** *Use 4 cups sliced nectarines and 2 cups blueberries in the filling.*
- **Apple Crisp:** *Instead of peaches, use 6 cups sliced apples. Add ½ tsp nutmeg.*
- **Strawberry Rhubarb Crisp:** *Instead of peaches, use 2 cups sliced strawberries and 4 cups fresh or frozen (thawed) rhubarb, cut in ½-inch pieces. Increase sugar in filling to ⅔ cup. Add 1 tsp grated orange zest.*

Strawberry and Banana Frozen Yogurt

For maximum flavor, use very ripe fruit for this recipe. Perfect for breakfast, snacks, or dessert.

1 pint very ripe strawberries, hulled (or 2 cups unsweetened frozen berries)
3 very ripe medium bananas, peeled
½ cup non-fat yogurt
1–2 tbsp honey (to taste)

1. Cut fruit into 1-inch pieces. Arrange in a single layer on a baking sheet and freeze for 2 or 3 hours, until firm. (Fruit can be frozen for several weeks in plastic storage bags.)
2. Place the processor bowl and Steel Knife into the freezer for 15 to 20 minutes. Combine all ingredients in chilled processor bowl. Process with quick on/offs to start, then let machine run until mixture is smooth. (If you have a small processor, do this in 2 batches.) Serve immediately, or transfer mixture to a serving bowl and freeze for up to ½ hour before serving.

Yield: 6 servings.

91 calories per serving, 0.5 g fat (0.1 g saturated), trace cholesterol, 2 g protein, 22 g carbohydrate, 17 mg sodium, 371 mg potassium, trace iron, 3 g fiber, 52 mg calcium.

■ HOMEMADE BREADS

The following breads taste so good, you won't believe they're low GI!

Fat-Free Sourdough Bread
Guilt-free and fabulous!

> 1 pkg active dry yeast
> 1½ cups lukewarm water (110°F)
> 1 cup Sourdough Starter (see page 62) at room temperature
> 5½–6 cups all-purpose flour
> 2 tsp salt
> 1 tbsp sugar
> ½ tsp baking soda

1. In a large bowl, sprinkle yeast over water. Let stand for 5 minutes, then stir to dissolve. Add Sourdough Starter, 2 cups flour, salt and sugar. Stir well. In another bowl, mix 3 cups flour with baking soda. Add to flour/yeast mixture along with enough of the remaining flour to make a stiff dough. Turn dough out onto a lightly floured surface. Knead until smooth and elastic, about 5 to 7 minutes. Add more flour as needed to prevent dough from sticking.

2. Shape dough into a ball and place it in a lightly greased bowl. Cover and let rise in a warm place for 1 to 1½ hours, until doubled. Punch down and divide in half. Cover and let rest for 10 minutes.

3. Shape dough into 2 round or baguette-shaped loaves and place them several inches apart on a lightly greased large baking sheet. With a sharp knife, make several diagonal slashes across the top of each loaf. (Round breads also look terrific if you make a tic-tac-toe design.) Cover and let rise until doubled, about 1 to 1½ hours. Dust tops lightly with a little flour, if desired.

4. Preheat oven to 375°F. Bake loaves for 35 to 40 minutes, or until bread sounds hollow when tapped with your fingertips. If desired, brush tops of breads with a little water 5 minutes before the end of baking. (This makes a crisp crust.) Remove bread from oven and cool completely.

Yield: 2 loaves (16 slices per loaf). These freeze well.

89 calories per slice, 0.2 g fat (0 g saturated), 0 mg cholesterol, 3 g protein, 19 g carbohydrate, 166 mg sodium, 31 mg potassium, 1 mg iron, <1 g fiber, 4 mg calcium.

Variation:

-   ***Whole-Wheat Sourdough Bread:*** *Replace 2 cups of all-purpose flour with whole-wheat flour in above recipe. Add 2 tbsp molasses and 2 tsp canola oil to yeast mixture along with starter.*

Maurice's Cranberry Bread (Bread Machine Method)

My friend Maurice Borts is an expert bread machine baker who enjoys creating unusual breads. The rolled oats add soluble fiber to lower the GI! Fruit loaves are usually medium GI otherwise.

> 1 cup water (room temperature)
> 2 tbsp canola oil
> 2 tbsp honey or sugar
> ¾ tsp salt
> ½ cup rolled oats
> ½ cup whole-wheat flour
> 2 cups bread flour
> 1½ tsp bread machine yeast
> ½–¾ cup dried cranberries (to taste)

1. Place all the ingredients (except cranberries) in baking pan of the bread machine in the order given. Select the whole-grain cycle or basic bread cycle. Add cranberries 5 minutes before the end of the kneading cycle (generally when the machine beeps to add additional ingredients). Using oven mitts, remove bread immediately after the bake cycle is finished to prevent crust from getting soggy. Cool bread on a rack. Fill pan immediately with lukewarm water and let soak for easier cleanup.

Yield: 1½-pound loaf (12 or less servings). This is addictive. Bread freezes well if there's any left!

160 calories per slice, 3 g fat (0.3 g saturated), 0 mg cholesterol, 4 g protein, 29 g carbohydrate, 147 mg sodium, 69 mg potassium, 2 mg iron, 2 g fiber, 8 mg calcium.

Oatmeal Wheat Germ Bread

1 cup rolled oats
2 cups boiling water
1 tsp sugar
½ cup lukewarm water (about 110°F)
1 pkg active dry yeast
¼ cup molasses
¼ cup maple syrup
2 tsp salt
2 tsp canola oil
3 cups all-purpose or bread flour
1½ cups whole-wheat flour
½ cup wheat germ
1 egg white beaten with 1 tbsp cold water

1. Place oats in a large mixing bowl. Pour boiling water over oats and let stand for 20 minutes. Dissolve sugar in ½ cup lukewarm water. Add yeast and let stand for 10 minutes. Stir to dissolve. Add yeast mixture to oats along with molasses, maple syrup, salt and oil. Slowly stir in flours and wheat germ; mix well. Transfer dough to a floured surface and knead for 3 or 4 minutes.
2. Place in a lightly greased large bowl, cover and let rise in a warm place for 1½ hours. Punch down. Shape into 2 loaves; place in sprayed loaf pans. Cover and let rise until doubled, about 1 hour. Brush with egg white mixture. Preheat oven to 375°F. Bake for 40 to 45 minutes, until golden. When done, loaves will pull away from sides of pans. Remove from pans and cool on racks.

Yield: 2 loaves (32 slices). These freeze well.

93 calories per slice (1/16 loaf), 0.8 g fat (0.1 g saturated), 0 mg cholesterol, 3 g protein, 19 g carbohydrate, 150 mg sodium, 103 mg potassium, 1 mg iron, 2 g fiber, 13 mg calcium.

Sourdough Rye Bread

1 pkg active dry yeast
1½ cups lukewarm water (110°F)
1 cup Sourdough Starter (see page 62) at room temperature
2 cups rye flour
2 tsp salt
2 tbsp sugar
2 tsp canola oil
1 tbsp molasses
1 tbsp caraway seeds
3 cups bread flour (approximately)
½ tsp baking soda
2–3 tbsp cornmeal
1 egg white, lightly beaten

1. In a large bowl, sprinkle yeast over water. Let stand for 5 minutes, then stir to dissolve. Add Sourdough Starter, rye flour, salt, sugar, oil and molasses. Stir well. Mix 2 cups of bread flour (or all-purpose flour) with baking soda. Add to flour/yeast mixture along with enough of the remaining flour to make a stiff dough. Turn dough out onto a lightly floured surface. Knead until smooth and elastic, about 6 to 8 minutes. Add additional flour as needed to prevent dough from sticking.
2. Shape dough into a ball and place it in a lightly greased bowl. Cover and let rise in a warm place for 1 to 1½ hours, until doubled. Punch down. (If you have time, let dough rise once again, until doubled.) Divide dough in half. Cover and let rest for 10 minutes.

3. Shape dough into 2 long loaves and place them a few inches apart on a lightly greased large baking sheet that has been sprinkled with cornmeal. With a sharp knife, make 4 or 5 diagonal slashes across the top of each loaf. Cover and let rise until doubled, about 1 to 1½ hours. Brush loaves lightly with egg white.
4. Preheat oven to 375°F. Bake for 35 to 40 minutes, or until breads sound hollow when tapped with your fingertips. Remove from oven and cool completely.

Yield: 2 loaves (16 slices per loaf). These freeze well.

84 calories per slice, 0.6 g fat (0.1 g saturated), 0 mg cholesterol, 3 g protein, 17 g carbohydrate, 168 mg sodium, 44 mg potassium, <1 mg iron, 1 g fiber, 8 mg calcium.

Note:

- *Chef's Secret! If you use all-purpose flour instead of bread flour, your loaf may spread and flatten. That's because bread flour is higher in gluten than all-purpose flour and produces a better-shaped loaf. My bread expert Fred Hansen suggests that if you don't have bread flour you can use 11/2 cup rye flour and 31/2 cups all-purpose flour to make your dough. You'll end up with a lighter rye bread than the one above, but it will still be tasty.*

Sourdough Starter

1 pkg active dry yeast (1 tbsp)
2 cups lukewarm water (110°F)
2 cups all-purpose flour

1. In a large glass bowl or non-metal container, dissolve yeast in water. Add flour and stir thoroughly. Cover loosely and let stand at room

temperature for three days. The first day, starter will bubble up and quadruple in volume, then deflate. After three days, stir well. Cover and refrigerate until ready to use.

Yield: About 3 cups starter. Can be frozen.

289 calories per cup, 0.9 g fat (0.1 g saturated), 0 mg cholesterol, 9 g protein, 60 g carbohydrate, 7 mg sodium, 127 mg potassium, 4 mg iron, 3 g fiber, 16 mg calcium.

■ SPREADS

These spreads are low GI and low fat!

Better than Butter Spread

Thanks to food writer Marcy Goldman for inspiring this recipe. Although this spread is lower in fat and cholesterol than butter, it's still high in fat. You can also use as a topping for baked potatoes, steamed veggies or as a spread for toast or sandwiches. Don't use it for frying because it contains yogurt.

⅓ cup lightly salted butter
⅓ cup canola oil
⅓ cup non-fat yogurt

1. Combine all ingredients and blend until smooth. (It takes just moments in the food processor.)

Yield: 1 cup. Mixture keeps about a week in the refrigerator.

80 calories per tbsp, 8.8 g fat (2.8 g saturated), 11 mg cholesterol, trace protein, trace carbohydrate, 45 mg sodium, 15 mg potassium, 0 mg iron, 0 g fiber, 12 mg calcium.

Notes:
- *Butter or margarine? The debate continues! The fat in butter is mostly saturated. Saturated fats are presumed to raise blood cholesterol levels more than other types of fat. Stick margarines are hydrogenated. Hydrogenation creates high levels of trans-fatty acids. Soft non-hydrogenated margarines are a better choice because they contain no trans-fatty acids. Both butter and margarine can be incorporated into a healthy diet, but use them sparingly. Moderation is the key.*
- *Instead of using butter or margarine as a spread for your bread with lunch and dinner, you can dip that bread in olive oil (to which you've added coarse salt, freshly ground pepper, minced garlic, basil, oregano and thyme). But dip lightly, or your hips will spread!*

Date and Apple Mixture (also used as "charoset" for the Jewish holiday, Passover)

This makes a delicious jam-like spread for low GI breads and muffins.

3 tbsp almonds or walnuts
2 apples, peeled and cored
¾ cup pitted dates
1 tsp grated lemon zest, optional
2–3 tbsp honey or sugar
3–4 tbsp sweet red wine (to taste)
1 tsp cinnamon*
¼ tsp ground ginger, optional

1.   Toast nuts at 350°F for 10 minutes. Cool slightly. In the processor, chop nuts coarsely with quick on/off turns. Add remaining ingredients and pulse several times, until coarsely chopped.

Yield: About 2 cups. (Recipe can be doubled easily.)

26 calories per tbsp, 0.4 g fat (0 g saturated), 0 mg cholesterol, trace protein, 5 g carbohydrate, trace sodium, 37 mg potassium, trace iron, <1 g fiber, 3 mg calcium.

Prune Purée

Homemade Prune Purée makes a delicious fat-free spread on low GI bread or toast instead of jam. One cup of Prune Purée contains 304 calories and less than 1 gram of fat. One cup of butter contains 1,628 calories and 184 grams of fat. One cup of oil contains 1,927 calories and 218 grams of fat! This is also a fabulous fat substitute for use in baking! It's quick and easy to make, plus it's much cheaper than the commercial version. Prune Purée is packed with potassium and fiber.

> 2 cups pitted prunes (about 36)
> 1 cup hot water

1. Combine prunes and hot water in a bowl. Cover and let stand for 5 minutes, until plump. In a processor or blender, process prunes with water until smooth, about 1 minute. Scrape down sides of bowl several times.

Yield: About 2 cups. Store tightly covered in the fridge for up to 3 months, or freeze for 6 months.

20 calories per tbsp, 0 g fat (0 g saturated), 0 mg cholesterol, trace protein, 5 g carbohydrate, <1 mg sodium, 63 mg potassium, trace iron, <1 g fiber, 4 mg calcium.

304 calories per cup, 0.7 g fat (0.1 g saturated), 0 mg cholesterol, 3 g protein, 80 g carbohydrate, 8 mg sodium, 948 mg potassium, 3 mg iron, 12 g fiber, 67 mg calcium.

■ MUFFINS

Apple Streusel Oatmeal Muffins

One day I was rushed for time and baked my cake in muffin pans. These were the result!

1.	Prepare batter for Apple Streusel Oatmeal Cake as directed (see page 77). Place batter in paper-lined muffin pans. Bake at 375°F for 25 minutes.

Yield: 15 muffins.

195 calories per muffin, 4.6 g fat (0.6 g saturated), 14 mg cholesterol, 4 g protein, 36 g carbohydrate, 92 mg sodium, 172 mg potassium, 1 mg iron, 2 g fiber, 53 mg calcium.

Bran and Date Muffins

Moist, low in fat and high in flavor, these are guaranteed to be a regular at your house! Originally, I was making these marvelous muffins with ¼ cup oil, but discovered that they tasted even more delicious when I substituted Prune Purée (see under Spreads, and in the Desserts chapter) for part of the fat.

1½ cups natural bran or All-Bran cereal
2 tbsp canola oil
¾–1 cup dates, cut-up
¾ cup raisins, rinsed and drained
½ cup hot water
2 tbsp Prune Purée (see page 65) or unsweetened applesauce
2 egg whites (or 1 egg)
1 cup buttermilk or sour milk
2 tbsp molasses or honey
1¼ cups flour (whole-wheat or all-purpose)
⅓ cup sugar (brown or white)

1 tsp baking soda
½ tsp baking powder

1. Combine bran, oil, dates and raisins in a large mixing bowl. Pour hot water over mixture; let cool slightly. Stir in purée, egg whites, buttermilk and molasses. Add remaining ingredients and stir just enough to moisten dry ingredients. If you have time, let mixture stand for 20 to 30 minutes. (I usually do this while the oven is heating and I'm cleaning up.)
2. Preheat oven to 400°F. Line muffin pans with paper liners. Fill ¾-full with batter. Bake for 20 to 25 minutes, until nicely browned.

Yield: 1 dozen. These freeze well.

193 calories per muffin, 3.2 g fat (0.4 g saturated), <1 mg cholesterol, 5 g protein, 42 g carbohydrate, 227 mg sodium, 424 mg potassium, 2 mg iron, 5 g fiber, 67 mg calcium.

Notes:

- *Fiber Facts: Bran is available in 2 forms, unprocessed and processed. Just compare: ½ cup unprocessed natural wheat bran (e.g., Quaker brand) contains 14 grams of dietary fiber and ½ cup of All-Bran contains 10 grams, while ½ cup processed Bran Flakes contains only 3 grams of fiber.*
- *To cut dates up easily, dip scissors in flour first. This prevents sticking. (For variety, make one batch of muffins with raisins or dried apricots, and make another batch with dates.)*
- *I prefer to use Prune Purée in these muffins. It takes just moments to make, adds fiber and flavor, and keeps perfectly in the fridge for at least 3 months. Do try it! You can substitute unsweetened applesauce if it's more convenient. Either one is excellent.*
- *To make sour milk, mix 1 tbsp lemon juice or vinegar plus skim milk to equal 1 cup. For dairy-free recipes, substitute soy or rice milk plus lemon juice or vinegar.*

- *An alternative to sour milk or buttermilk in muffin and cake recipes is to mix ½ cup of non-fat yogurt with ½ cup of water.*
- *For even-sized muffins, scoop out batter with an ice cream scoop, or use a ½ cup dry measure.*

Variation:

- ***Lee's Ever-Ready Muffin Mixture:*** *Lee Stillinger, one of my enthusiastic students, loves this recipe so much she makes 4 times the original and stores the batter in the refrigerator in an airtight container (it keeps for about 3 weeks). That way, she can have fresh muffins whenever she's in the mood. (If you're not quite as enthusiastic, just double the recipe!)*

MUFFINFORMATION!

- Homemade muffins contain less fat and calories than most commercial mega-muffins. A muffin can be a little cake in disguise and may contain more than 500 calories, with 30 to 35 grams of fat!
- Substitute unsweetened applesauce or Prune Purée (see page 65) for half the fat in your favorite muffins.
- If you store an open box of baking soda in the fridge to absorb odors, don't use it for baking.
- Batters made only with baking soda have to be baked right away because they release all their leavening when mixed with liquid. Baking soda should be mixed together with dry ingredients.
- Muffin batters made with baking powder can be stored tightly covered in the refrigerator for 2 or 3 days before baking. This is because baking powder releases part of its leavening when it comes in contact with liquid, then releases the remainder when exposed to oven heat.
- To test if baking powder is still active, stir 1 tsp baking powder into ½ cup hot water. If it fizzes, it's good. Baking powder keeps about a year stored in a dry place in a tightly closed container.
- For variety, add dried cherries, cranberries, blueberries or strawberries to muffin batters.

- Over-mixing makes muffins heavy and full of tunnels. If using a processor, use quick on/offs to mix the dry and wet ingredients together. If mixing by hand, 15 to 20 strokes is usually enough, just until flour disappears. Mixture will be lumpy rather than smooth.
- Lining muffin pans with paper liners makes for easy removal and cleanup. Muffins made with little or no fat may stick to the paper liners, so you may prefer to use non-stick spray.
- Muffin compartments should be filled ¾-full before baking. A half-cup measure or ice cream scoop can be used for measuring batter into compartments of muffin pan.
- Overfilling causes batter to spill onto top of the pan, producing muffins with overhanging tops. Muffins will be harder to remove, plus the pan will require scrubbing.
- Muffins should be baked in a preheated oven at 375°F to 400°F on the center rack.
- When done, tops of muffins will be golden brown and will spring back when lightly touched. A cake tester inserted into the center of the muffin should come out clean.
- Miniatures: Bake 12 to 15 minutes at 375°F. Three minis equal one regular muffin.
- Jumbos: Bake 25 to 30 minutes at 375°F. One jumbo muffin equals 1½ regular muffins.
- Mushroom Cap Muffins: These are baked in a special pan with an extra rim around the edge of each compartment to handle the extra batter. (Pans are available in bakery supply houses or specialty kitchen boutiques.) Fill each compartment of sprayed or greased pans just to the top, but don't let batter overflow into the rims. As the batter rises, it will flow into the rims.
- Muffin Tops: These are baked in special pans with shallow, round compartments. You end up with crusty muffin tops, the favorite part of the muffin for many people!

- Muffin Loaf: Instead of using a muffin pan, line a 9 x 5-inch loaf pan with aluminum foil and spray with non-stick spray. Pour muffin batter into prepared pan. Bake loaf in a preheated 350°F oven for 45 to 55 minutes, or until a cake tester inserted comes out clean. Thanks to Carolyn Melmed for the terrific idea! (While the loaf bakes, I try to go out for a brisk walk!)
- Muffin batter can also be baked in a cake pan. This is easier than trying to divide the batter evenly among the compartments of your muffin pan, and also saves on cleaning up those inevitable spills around the edges! The batter for 12 muffins can be baked in a 7 x 11-inch cake pan. Your baking time will be 35 to 45 minutes at 350°F. When cooled, cut into squares to serve.
- One regular-size muffin takes 20 to 25 seconds on HIGH to defrost in the microwave.

Bran and Honey Muffins

Cathy Ternan, my exercise partner, special friend and proofreader, shared this excellent do-ahead muffin recipe with me. I replaced part of the honey with molasses and used applesauce to replace part of the fat in these tender, tasty muffins. They're not too sweet and are packed with fiber and flavor.

6 cups natural bran, divided
1¾ cups boiling water
½ cup canola oil
1¾ cups honey
¼ cup molasses
½ cup unsweetened applesauce
4 eggs (or 2 eggs plus 4 egg whites)
4 cups buttermilk
5 cups whole-wheat flour
5 tsp baking soda

1 tsp salt
1 tbsp cinnamon*
2 cups raisins, rinsed and drained

1. Place 2 cups of bran in a very large mixing bowl or storage container. Pour boiling water over bran, stir well to moisten and let mixture stand for about 5 minutes.
2. Add oil, honey, molasses, applesauce, eggs, buttermilk and remaining bran to bowl. Stir to combine. Sift in flour, baking soda and salt. Mix in cinnamon and raisins. Batter will keep for up to 6 weeks in the refrigerator. Bake as many muffins as needed.
3. Preheat oven to 375°F. Fill paper-lined muffin cups ¾-full with batter. Bake for 20 to 25 minutes, until nicely browned.

Yield: About 4 dozen. These freeze well.

164 calories per muffin, 3.6 g fat (0.5 g saturated), 18 mg cholesterol, 4 g protein, 33 g carbohydrate, 266 mg sodium, 275 mg potassium, 2 mg iron, 4 g fiber, 45 mg calcium.

Notes:

- *Quaker Oats makes natural wheat bran (in a green box), or you can buy it in bulk. Substitute all or part All-Bran cereal if you're short of natural bran.*
- *Optional at baking time: Add chopped dates, apples, chocolate chips, nuts, etc. to batter.*

Variation:

- ***Oatmeal Bran Muffins:*** *Follow recipe above, but use 4 cups of wheat bran and 2 cups of rolled oats. Replace the honey with 2 cups of firmly packed brown sugar.*

Carolyn's Thin Muffin Loaf

Carolyn Melmed walked side by side with me on the treadmill most mornings in our quest for thinness and health! She shared her delicious recipe for bran muffins, which she bakes as a loaf. I revised it slightly, reducing fat and sugar without a loss in flavor or moistness. Enjoy without the guilt!

2 cups All-Bran or natural bran cereal
1¾ cup skim milk
½ cup orange juice
2 eggs (or 1 egg plus 2 egg whites)
¼ cup canola oil
½ cup unsweetened applesauce (or Prune Purée, page 65)
2 tsp vanilla
1 cup flour plus 1 cup whole-wheat flour (or 2 cups all-purpose flour)
2 tsp baking powder
2 tsp baking soda
1 cup brown sugar, packed
1 cup raisins, rinsed and drained

1. Preheat oven to 350°F. Line two 9 x 5 x 3-inch loaf pans completely with aluminum foil. Spray with non-stick spray. Measure bran into a large bowl. Add milk, orange juice, eggs, oil, applesauce and vanilla. Let stand for 5 minutes. Add remaining ingredients to bran mixture. Mix just until blended. Do not over-mix.

2. Pour mixture into prepared pans. Bake at 350°F for 50 to 55 minutes, or until a cake tester inserted into the center of the loaf comes out clean. Cool 10 minutes. Remove from pans.

Yield: 2 loaves (24 slices). These loaves freeze beautifully. If well wrapped, they'll stay fresh for 3 or 4 days at room temperature.

145 calories per slice, 3.1 g fat (0.4 g saturated), 18 mg cholesterol, 4 g protein, 29 g carbohydrate, 246 mg sodium, 240 mg potassium, 2 mg iron, 4 g fiber, 66 mg calcium.

Notes:
- *Lighter Bake, which is a fat substitute made from fruit purée, works beautifully in this recipe.*
- *When I was in the middle of preparing to move to Toronto, I packed most of my baking pans. All that was left in my kitchen was one lonely 9 x 13-inch rectangular pan. Not to worry! I just made one big muffin cake! (Baking time is about 5 minutes less if you bake the batter in a cake pan.)*

Carrot Muffins

1. Prepare Moist 'n Luscious Carrot Cake (see under Cakes) as directed. Pour batter into sprayed muffin pans and bake at 375°F for 20 to 25 minutes.

Yield: 18 muffins.

193 calories per muffin, 3 g fat (0.3 g saturated), 12 mg cholesterol, 3 g protein, 40 g carbohydrate, 180 mg sodium, 173 mg potassium, 1 mg iron, 2 g fiber, 19 mg calcium.

Mary's Best Bran-ana Bread

Low in fat, high in flavor! I reduced the fat by half from Mary Goldwater's yummy recipe. I'm glad she shared it because it's become one of my absolute favorites. Also refer to Going Bananas (see page 74).

> 2 tbsp canola oil
> 1 cup sugar
> 1 egg plus 2 egg whites (or 2 eggs)

1 tsp vanilla
1 cup All-Bran cereal
2 tbsp water or skim milk
3 very ripe bananas (1½ cups mashed)
1½ cups flour (part whole-wheat can be used)
⅛ tsp salt
2 tsp baking powder
½ tsp baking soda

1. Preheat oven to 350°F. Spray a 9 x 5-inch loaf pan. In the processor or a large bowl, beat oil, sugar, egg, egg whites and vanilla. Add bran; mix well. Add bananas and water and beat until smooth. Add dry ingredients and mix just until blended. Pour batter into prepared pan and bake at 350°F for 1 hour. A cake tester should come out dry.

Yield: 1 loaf (12 slices). Freezes well.

196 calories per slice, 3.1 g fat (0.4 g saturated), 18 mg cholesterol, 4 g protein, 41 g carbohydrate, 263 mg sodium, 230 mg potassium, 2 mg iron, 4 g fiber, 58 mg calcium.

GOING BANANAS?
- *Banana Muffins:* Follow recipe for Banana Bread above, but bake batter in muffin pans. You'll get 16 muffins. (Fill the empty muffin compartments with water.) Bake at 375°F for 20 to 25 minutes. One muffin contains 170 calories, 4.1 grams fat (0.4 grams saturated), 14 milligrams cholesterol and 31 grams carbohydrate.
- *Banana Blueberry Muffins:* 1½ cups of fresh or frozen blueberries (do not thaw if frozen) can be added to the batter. Place batter in paper-lined or sprayed muffin tins. Place 6 or 8 blueberries on top of each muffin and press gently into batter. (This method prevents streaking.) Bake muffins at 375°F for 20 to 25 minutes. Blueberries are a great source of fiber!

(One muffin contains 178 calories and 2 grams fiber.)

- If you have a lot of ripe bananas on hand and don't have time to bake, don't bother peeling and mashing them. Just put the bananas in a plastic freezer bag and freeze them until needed. When you do have time to bake, thaw them slightly (about 10 minutes at room temperature). Peel and cut into chunks. Process bananas with the Steel Knife of the processor until smooth.
- If you're in a hurry, put frozen banana under hot water for 30 seconds, or defrost for 20 seconds on HIGH in the microwave. Cut away the peel with a sharp paring knife.
- Another suggestion for using up ripe bananas is to peel them, then mash and freeze them in containers holding the exact amount you need for your favorite recipe. Thaw before using.
- When bananas are on sale, buy a bunch and freeze them, using any of the methods above.
- Make some Banana Smoothies (see page 52) or Strawberry and Banana Frozen Yogurt (see page 56)!

Rozie's Magical Carrot Muffins
These versatile muffins will disappear like magic!

1½ cups whole-wheat flour (all-purpose flour can replace part of the flour)

⅛ tsp salt

1½ tsp baking soda

1 tsp cinnamon*

¾ cup wheat bran

¾ cup oat bran

1 cup grated carrots (about 3 medium)

1 egg plus 2 egg whites (or 2 eggs)

3 tbsp canola oil

1½ cups orange juice, skim milk or yogurt

2 tbsp lemon juice

⅔ cup maple syrup or honey

¾ cup raisins or cut-up prunes (or ½ cup mini chocolate chips)

1. Preheat oven to 375°F. Combine dry ingredients and blend well. Add carrots, egg, egg whites and oil. Mix until blended. Add orange juice, lemon juice, maple syrup and raisins (or chocolate chips). Mix just until blended. Line muffin cups with paper liners. Fill ¾-full with batter. Bake at 375°F for 20 to 25 minutes, until golden brown.

Yield: 18 muffins. These freeze well.

145 calories per muffin, 3.3 g fat (0.4 g saturated), 14 mg cholesterol, 4 g protein, 29 g carbohydrate, 166 mg sodium, 251 mg potassium, 1 mg iron, 3 g fiber, 28 mg calcium.

Wheat Germ Bran Muffins

Wheat germ should be stored in the refrigerator to prevent it from becoming rancid.

3 tbsp tub margarine or canola oil

½ cup brown sugar, packed

¼ cup molasses

2 eggs (or 1 egg plus 2 egg whites)

1 cup skim milk

1½ cups natural bran

¼ cup wheat germ

½ cup all-purpose flour

½ cup whole-wheat flour

1½ tsp baking powder

½ tsp baking soda

¾ cup raisins, rinsed and drained (or chopped dates)

1 tbsp grated orange zest

1. Preheat oven to 400°F. Beat margarine with brown sugar, molasses and eggs until well blended, about 2 or 3 minutes. Add milk and bran; blend well. Add wheat germ, flours, baking powder and soda. Mix just until smooth. Stir in raisins and orange zest. Spoon the batter into paper-lined muffin cups, filling them about ¾-full. Bake at 400°F for 20 to 25 minutes, until golden brown.

Yield: 12 muffins. These freeze well.

197 calories per muffin, 4.6 g fat (1 g saturated), 36 mg cholesterol, 5 g protein, 38 g carbohydrate, 223 mg sodium, 407 mg potassium, 3 mg iron, 4 g fiber, 101 mg calcium.

Variation:

- **Bran and Prune Muffins:** *Follow recipe for Wheat Germ Bran Muffins (above), but substitute 1 cup of cut-up pitted prunes for raisins. (Dip your scissors in flour first to cut prunes.)*

■ CAKES FOR BREAKFAST

These two cakes make wonderful breakfasts, snacks or desserts!

Apple Streusel Oatmeal Cake

A delicious oatmeal and apple cake, topped with a mixture like those used on fruit crisps. Pleasure without guilt!

Topping:
¼ cup flour
½ cup rolled oats
1 tsp cinnamon*
1 tbsp tub margarine or canola oil
1 tbsp water
¼ cup brown sugar, packed

Batter:

1 cup rolled oats
¾ cup non-fat yogurt
¼ cup unsweetened applesauce
2 large apples, peeled and cored
1 egg plus 1 egg white
1 cup brown sugar, firmly packed
3 tbsp canola oil
1 cup flour
1 tsp baking powder
½ tsp baking soda
1 tsp cinnamon*

1. Preheat oven to 350°F. Spray a 7 x 11-inch oblong pan with non-stick spray. In a bowl, mix topping ingredients together until crumbly. Set aside.
2. In another bowl, combine oats, yogurt and applesauce; mix well. Let stand until softened, about 3 or 4 minutes. Grate or chop apples; set aside. In the processor, combine egg, egg white, brown sugar and 3 tbsp oil and beat until well mixed, about 2 to 3 minutes. Add oats/yogurt mixture and mix just until blended. Add flour, baking powder, soda and cinnamon. Mix briefly, just enough to moisten the flour mixture. Gently mix in apples.
3. Pour batter into pan. Sprinkle evenly with crumb topping. Bake at 350°F for 45 to 50 minutes. A toothpick inserted into the center of the loaf should come out without any batter clinging to it.

Yield: 15 servings. Freezes well.

195 calories per serving, 4.6 g fat (0.6 g saturated), 14 mg cholesterol, 4 g protein, 36 g carbohydrate, 92 mg sodium, 172 mg potassium, 1 mg iron, 2 g fiber, 53 mg calcium.

Moist 'n Luscious Carrot Cake

Dave Horan's favorite! You won't believe it's low fat. Most low-fat carrot cakes include buttermilk or yogurt, but I was determined to create a dairy-free cake. My testers loved the results. Icing will raise the GI value of this cake, but if you must have icing on your cake, combine ½ cup icing sugar to 250 milliliters (1 cup) extra-light cream cheese.

>   3 cups grated carrots (6–8 carrots)
>   1 egg plus 2 egg whites (or 2 eggs)
>   3 tbsp canola oil
>   1¾ cups sugar
>   2 tsp vanilla
>   ¾ cup unsweetened applesauce
>   2½ cups flour (I use half whole-wheat flour)
>   1½ tsp baking powder
>   1½ tsp baking soda
>   1 tbsp cinnamon*
>   ¼ tsp salt
>   2 tbsp wheat germ
>   ½ cup raisins or mini chocolate chips

1. Preheat oven to 350°F. Spray a 9 x 13-inch baking pan with non-stick spray. Grate carrots, measure 3 cups and set aside. Beat egg, egg whites, oil, sugar, vanilla and applesauce. Beat until light, about 2 to 3 minutes. Add grated carrots and mix well. Combine flour, baking powder, baking soda, cinnamon, salt and wheat germ. Add to batter and mix just until flour disappears. Stir in raisins or chocolate chips. Pour batter into prepared pan. Bake at 350°F for 45 to 50 minutes, or until a toothpick inserted into the center of the cake comes out with no batter clinging to it.

Yield: 24 servings. Freezes well.

144 calories per serving (without frosting), 2.2 g fat (0.2 g saturated), 9 mg cholesterol, 3 g protein, 30 g carbohydrate, 135 mg sodium, 130 mg potassium, <1 mg iron, 2 g fiber, 14 mg calcium.

Cinnamon Note

*A 2003 study published in *Diabetes Care* by Khan et al. has shown that taking less than a teaspoon of cinnamon a day may produce an approximately 20% drop in blood sugar, as well as lower cholesterol and triglycerides.

CHAPTER FIVE

LUNCHES

WHAT'S INSIDE

■ SOUPS

Soup and a salad make the perfect low GI lunch!

Bean, Barley and Sweet Potato Soup

1 cup dried white beans (navy or pea)
3 cups cold water
2 tsp canola or olive oil
2 large onions, peeled and chopped
4 stalks celery, trimmed and chopped
2 zucchini, chopped (optional)
1 red pepper, chopped (optional)
8 cups chicken broth or hot water
4 carrots, sliced
1 sweet potato, peeled and chopped
½ cup pearl barley, rinsed and drained
½ tsp pepper
1 tsp dried basil
salt, to taste

1. Soak beans in water overnight. Drain and rinse well. Discard soaking water. Heat oil on medium heat in a large heavy-bottomed soup pot. Sauté onions and celery for 5 minutes, until golden. Add zucchini and red pepper and cook 5 minutes longer. Add a little water if needed to prevent burning. Add remaining ingredients except salt. Bring to a boil. Reduce heat, cover partially and simmer for 2 hours, stirring occasionally. If soup is too thick, add a little water. Add salt; season to taste.

Yield: 10 to 12 servings. Reheats and/or freezes well.

173 calories per serving, 1.3 g fat (0.2 g saturated), 0 mg cholesterol, 12 g protein, 29 g carbohydrate, 175 mg sodium, 498 mg potassium, 4 mg iron, 7 g fiber, 90 mg calcium.

Get Skinny Cabbage Soup

This is a version of the famous "miracle cabbage soup" that people eat in hopes of getting slim quickly.

> 2 green peppers
> 1 bunch of celery
> 1 bunch of green onions
> 1 medium head of cabbage
> 28 oz (796 ml) canned crushed tomatoes
> 19 oz (540 ml) V-8 vegetable juice
> 1 pkg dry onion soup mix (4-serving size)

1. Chop vegetables. Combine all ingredients in a large pot, adding water to cover veggies. Bring to a boil; cook for 10 minutes. Reduce heat and simmer partially covered for 25 minutes.

Yield: 12 servings. Reheats and/or freezes well.

61 calories per serving, 0.8 g fat (0.1 g saturated), 0 mg cholesterol, 3 g protein, 13 g carbohydrate, 547 mg sodium, 468 mg potassium, 1 mg iron, 5 g fiber, 76 mg calcium.

Notes and Variations:
- *Add a handful of chopped mushrooms to the pot along with the chopped vegetables and cook as directed. The soaking water from dried mushrooms can also be added.*
- *For a sweet and sour taste, add a squeeze of lemon juice and a little low GI sweetener.*
- *If desired, add a splash of low-cal cranberry juice to the cooked soup.*
- *Just before the soup is done, add 2 cups of washed, chopped spinach or Swiss chard.*

Greek-Style Lentil Soup

Easy and healthy! Although it takes about the same amount of time to microwave this soup as to cook it on top of the stove, it never sticks to the bottom
of the pot when you microwave it. Your food processor will chop the
vegetables 1-2-3.

> 1 large onion, chopped
> 4 cloves garlic, minced
> 1 tbsp olive or canola oil
> 1 cup brown or red lentils, rinsed and drained
> 1 stalk celery, chopped
> 28 oz (796 ml) can tomatoes (or 5 to 6 fresh ripe tomatoes, chopped)
> 5 cups water (approximately)
> 1 bay leaf
> 1 ½ tsp salt (to taste)
> ½ tsp pepper
> 1 tsp dried basil or dill (or 1 tbsp fresh)
> juice of half a lemon (1½ tbsp)
> ¼ cup parsley, minced

- *Microwave Method:* In a 3-quart microsafe pot, combine onion, garlic
  and oil. Microwave uncovered on HIGH for 4 minutes. Add remaining
  ingredients except lemon juice and parsley; mix well. Microwave covered
  on HIGH for 1 hour, until lentils are tender. Stir once or twice during
  cooking. If boiling too much, reduce power to MEDIUM (50%). If too
  thick, add some boiling water. Add lemon juice. Adjust seasonings to
  taste. Let stand at least 10 minutes to allow flavors to blend. Discard bay
  leaf. Garnish with parsley.
- *Conventional Method:* Heat oil in a large soup pot. Add onions and sauté
  on medium heat until golden, about 4 or 5 minutes. Add garlic and sauté
  2 or 3 minutes longer. Add 2 or 3 tablespoons of water if vegetables begin
  to stick. Add remaining ingredients except lemon juice and parsley. Bring

to a boil, reduce heat and simmer 1 hour, until lentils are tender, stirring occasionally. Thin with a little hot water if too thick. Add lemon juice. Adjust seasonings to taste. Discard bay leaf. Garnish with parsley.

Yield: 8 to 10 servings. Tastes even better the next day! Freezes well.

120 calories per serving, 2.1 g fat (0.3 g saturated), 0 mg cholesterol, 7 g protein, 20 g carbohydrate, 603 mg sodium, 533 mg potassium, 3 mg iron, 7 g fiber, 63 mg calcium.

Variations:

- *For more fiber, add 2 or 3 carrots, coarsely chopped, to the sautéed onions. Proceed as directed. Sprinkle with a little grated Parmesan cheese. For a Middle Eastern flavor, substitute coriander (cilantro) for basil or dill.*
- *Lentil, Vegetable and Barley Soup: Prepare Greek-Style Lentil Soup as directed above, but add 3 carrots and 1 zucchini, coarsely chopped, to the sautéed vegetables. Also add ⅓ cup barley, which has been rinsed and drained. Then continue as directed. If cooked soup is too thick, add a little water or vegetable stock.*

Green Split Pea and Barley Soup

For a delicious smoky flavor, add the cut-up carcass of a smoked turkey along with the barley!

2 cups green split peas, rinsed and drained
3 carrots, chopped
3–4 stalks celery, chopped
1 medium onion, chopped
12 cups water, chicken or vegetable broth
½ cup pearl barley, rinsed and drained
1 bay leaf
salt and pepper, to taste

2 cloves crushed garlic, if desired
2 tsp canola oil
2 medium onions, chopped
¼ cup chopped fresh dill

1. In a large soup pot, combine split peas, carrots, celery and 1 onion with water. Bring to a boil. Stir in barley, bay leaf and garlic, if using. Reduce heat and simmer partly covered for 1½ to 2 hours. Stir occasionally. Add salt and pepper to taste. In a non-stick skillet, heat oil. Sauté the remaining 2 onions on medium heat until well browned, about 6 to 8 minutes. Add onions to soup along with dill. Simmer soup 5 to 10 minutes longer. Discard bay leaf (and turkey carcass, if using).

Yield: 12 servings. Reheats and/or freezes well. If soup gets thick, add a little water or broth.

152 calories per serving, 1.3 g fat (0.1 g saturated), 0 mg cholesterol, 8 g protein, 28 g carbohydrate, 31 mg sodium, 427 mg potassium, 2 mg iron, 9 g fiber, 34 mg calcium.

New-Wave Gazpacho (Salad Soup)

Now you can sip your salad! So refreshing, so healthy, so tasty.

1 green and 1 red pepper
1 English cucumber, peeled
2 stalks celery
5–6 large, firm, ripe tomatoes
4 green onions
4 cloves garlic, crushed
2 tbsp each fresh dill and basil, minced
19 oz can (540 ml) tomato juice
2 cups vegetable broth
1 tbsp olive oil (extra-virgin is best)

3 tbsp fresh lemon juice (juice of a lemon)
salt and freshly ground pepper, to taste
6–8 drops Tabasco sauce

1. Chop the peppers, cucumber, celery, tomatoes and green onions.
    Combine together in a large bowl with garlic, dill and basil. Add remaining ingredients and mix well. Chill before serving.

Yield: 7 to 8 servings (about 10 cups). Soup will keep 2 or 3 days in the refrigerator.

84 calories per serving, 2.8 g fat (0.4 g saturated), 0 mg cholesterol, 3 g protein, 15 g carbohydrate, 610 mg sodium, 646 mg potassium, 2 mg iron, 3 g fiber, 37 mg calcium.

Variation:
*   ***Gazpacho Rosa:*** *Stir ⅓ cup non-fat yogurt or sour cream into each cup of soup.*

Red Lentil, Vegetable and Barley Soup

1 tbsp olive or canola oil
3 large onions, chopped
4 cloves garlic, minced
¼ cup fresh parsley, minced
4 stalks celery, chopped
6 carrots, coarsely chopped
1 large sweet potato, peeled and chopped
2 zucchini, ends trimmed, chopped
10 cups water, chicken or vegetable broth
1½ cups red lentils, rinsed and drained
½ cup pearl barley, rinsed and drained
1 tbsp salt (or to taste)
½ tsp pepper
1 tsp dried basil (or 1 tbsp fresh)
2 tbsp fresh dill, minced

1. Heat oil in a large soup pot. Add garlic and onions. Sauté on medium heat until golden, about 5 to 7 minutes. Add a little water if vegetables begin to stick. Add remaining ingredients. Bring to a boil, reduce heat and simmer partly covered for 1 hour, or until barley is tender. Stir occasionally. Thin with a little water if soup is too thick. Adjust seasonings to taste.

Yield: 12 servings. Soup freezes and/or reheats well.

169 calories per serving, 1.7 g fat (0.3 g saturated), 0 mg cholesterol, 8 g protein, 32 g carbohydrate, 629 mg sodium, 530 mg potassium, 3 mg iron, 10 g fiber, 55 mg calcium.

Red Lentil, Zucchini and Couscous Soup

1 large onion, chopped
1 stalk celery, chopped
2 tsp olive oil
3–4 carrots, grated
2 medium zucchini, grated
1 cup red lentils, picked over, rinsed and drained
6 cups water or vegetable broth (about)
2 tsp salt (or to taste)
½ tsp pepper
½ tsp dried basil
1/3 cup couscous

1. Onions and celery can be chopped in the processor, using quick on/off turns. Heat oil in a 5-quart soup pot. Add onions and celery. Sauté on medium-high heat for 5 to 7 minutes, or until golden. If vegetables begin to stick, add a tablespoon or two of water.

2. Meanwhile, grate carrots and zucchini. Add all ingredients except couscous to pot. Bring to a boil. Reduce heat and simmer partially covered for 45 minutes, stirring occasionally. Add couscous and simmer 10 minutes longer. If soup is too thick, thin with a little water. Adjust seasonings to taste.

Yield: 8 servings. Freezes well.

134 calories per serving, 1.5 g fat (0.2 g saturated), 0 mg cholesterol, 8 g protein, 24 g carbohydrate, 612 mg sodium, 430 mg potassium, 3 mg iron, 8 g fiber, 39 mg calcium.

Spinach and Rhubarb Soup (a.k.a. "Mock Shaav")

Miriam Bercovitz shared this great recipe! The Eastern European soup, Shaav, is usually made with sorrel, which can be expensive.

> 10-oz pkg (300 g) frozen chopped spinach
> ½ lb (250 g/2 cups) frozen rhubarb (or 1 lb fresh rhubarb)
> 6½ cups water
> 2 tsp salt, or to taste
> 1 egg, lightly beaten
> ½ cup non-fat yogurt or sour cream

1. Combine spinach, rhubarb, 6 cups water and salt in a large saucepan. Cook on high heat, breaking up spinach and rhubarb with a spoon. Once soup boils, cook uncovered on medium for 5 minutes. Combine egg and ½ cup cold water in a bowl. Gradually add hot soup a spoonful at a time to egg mixture (1½ cups soup in total). Stir egg mixture back into soup. Chill before serving. Serve cold with a dollop of yogurt or sour cream. Garnish with cucumbers, green onions and radishes.

Yield: 6 to 8 servings. Store in jars in the fridge for up to 10 days (without garnishes).

46 calories per serving, 1.1 g fat (0.3 g saturated), 36 mg cholesterol, 4 g protein, 6 g carbohydrate, 850 mg sodium, 244 mg potassium, 1 mg iron, 3 g fiber, 192 mg calcium.

Note:
- *Optional garnishes include chopped cucumbers, green onions and radishes.*

The Best Chicken Soup

I make my chicken soup with lots of carrots because they add wonderful flavor. Also, I love carrots! When I had pneumonia, my friend Doris Fink nursed me back to health by adding a red pepper to the soup. Since I did recover, I now use her trick when making chicken soup. I also add garlic and lots of dill. Chicken soup really is a marvelous cure for colds and flu, and it tastes terrific!

3 lb chicken (1.4 kg), cut up
8 cups water (approximately)
salt, to taste
½ tsp pepper
7–8 carrots
4 stalks celery
2 onions (or 1 onion and 1 leek)
1 red pepper, cored, seeded and cut up
2 cloves garlic
½ cup fresh dill sprigs (do not chop)

1. Trim excess fat from chicken. To remove excess salt from Kosher chicken, soak it in cold water for a half hour. Rinse and drain well. Place chicken in a narrow, deep soup pot. Add water. (It should cover the chicken completely.) Add salt and pepper. Bring to a boil. Remove scum

completely. Add carrots, celery, onions and red pepper. Cover partially simmer gently for 1 to 1½ hours. Add garlic and dill. Simmer soup 10 to 15 minutes longer. Adjust seasonings to taste.

2. Cool completely. Strain soup. Discard skin and fat from chicken. Discard all veggies except the carrots. Refrigerate soup overnight. Discard hardened fat from surface of soup.

Yield: 6 to 8 servings. Reheats and/or freezes well.

About 20 calories per cup of clear broth (without chicken), 1 g fat (0 g saturated), 1 mg cholesterol, 2 g protein, 3 g carbohydrate, 65 mg sodium, 20 mg calcium. (Note: clear, skimmed soup contains negligible calories.)

Notes and Variations:
- *Serve soup with noodles, orzo, kasha, Add a piece of carrot to each bowl, garnish with fresh dill.*
- *Serve boiled chicken as a main dish, or add pieces of cut-up chicken to the soup. Cooked chicken can be used for chicken salad, casseroles, or sandwiches.*
- *Some cooks add a piece of turnip, celery root, a few parsnips and/or parsley to the soup. It depends on what your mother added when she made her soup (or maybe not)!*
- *Jewish chicken soup is traditionally flavored with dill and the veggies are cooked in large chunks. French chefs add thyme and bay leaf to their soup, and they dice the vegetables neatly. That's very good chicken soup, but it's not Jewish chicken soup!*
- ***Turkey Broth:*** *Follow recipe for Chicken Soup, but use 4 to 5 pounds turkey bones, wings and backs.*

Vegetable Broth ("Almost Chicken Soup")

This recipe is a different version of vegetarian "chicken" soup.

> 2 large onions (or 1 onion and 1 leek, including about 2" of green top)
> 7–8 carrots
> 4 stalks celery
> 1 red pepper
> 1 cup mushrooms, optional
> 9 cups cold water
> salt, optional
> pepper, to taste
> 3 cloves garlic, peeled
> ½ cup fresh dill sprigs (do not chop)

1. Clean vegetables and cut them into large chunks. Place all ingredients except garlic and dill into a large soup pot. Water should cover vegetables by no more than 1 inch. Bring to a boil. Reduce heat, cover partially and simmer for 30 minutes.
2. Add garlic and dill and cook 10 minutes longer. Strain and serve with noodles, orzo (rice-shaped noodles), etc. Or use in recipes calling for vegetable broth.

Yield: About 8 cups. Clear broth contains negligible nutrients. Broth can be frozen for 3 or 4 months.

About 20 calories per cup, 1 g fat (0 g saturated), 0 mg cholesterol, 2 g protein, 3 g carbohydrate, 65 mg sodium, trace calcium.

■ SALADS AND DRESSINGS

Balsamic Salad Splash

An almost fat-free dressing. Perfect over salad greens.

> ¼ cup balsamic vinegar
> ¼ cup water
> ¼ cup honey
> ¼ tsp garlic powder
> 3–4 drops Tabasco sauce (to taste)
> 2 tsp olive or canola oil

1. Combine all ingredients in a jar; shake well. Refrigerate until needed. Shake well before serving.

Yield: About ¾ cup. Dressing can be stored in the refrigerator for up to a month.

28 calories per tbsp, 0.6 g fat (0.1 g saturated), 0 mg cholesterol, 0 g protein, 6 g carbohydrate, 2 mg sodium, 4 mg potassium, trace iron, 0 g fiber, 1 mg calcium.

Barley Salad with Honey Mustard Dressing

Barley is high in soluble fiber. Store it in a sealed jar in the pantry for at least 6 months.

> 3 cup lightly salted water
> 1 cup pearl or pot barley (if using pot barley, soak it overnight)
> 1 red pepper, chopped
> 4 green onions, chopped
> ½ cup Honey Mustard Dressing (see page 103)
> 2–3 tbsp fresh dill and/or basil, minced
> 2 tbsp toasted sunflower seeds, optional

1. Bring water to a boil. Add barley and simmer covered for 45 to 60 minutes, until tender. (Pearl barley takes 45 minutes to cook; pot barley takes about an hour.) Drain if necessary. Barley can be cooked in advance and refrigerated up to 24 hours. Combine chilled barley with remaining ingredients and toss to mix.

Yield: 6 servings. Leftovers will keep in the fridge for 3 days. Add a little lemon juice to moisten.

179 calories per serving, 4 g fat (0.6 g saturated), 0 mg cholesterol, 4 g protein, 34 g carbohydrate, 53 mg sodium, 152 mg potassium, 1 mg iron, 6 g fiber, 20 mg calcium.

Creamy Cole Slaw

This super slaw is virtually fat-free and high in fiber and potassium. Enjoy without guilt!

1 medium green cabbage (about 8 cups shredded)
6 green onions, chopped
3 stalks celery, chopped
1 green and 1 red pepper, chopped
3 carrots, grated
½ cup non-fat yogurt
½ cup non-fat or low-fat mayonnaise
½ cup ketchup or salsa
2 tbsp fresh chopped basil (or 1 tsp dried)
2 tbsp minced fresh dill
salt and pepper, to taste

1. Prepare vegetables. (You can do this quickly in the processor.) Combine veggies in a large bowl. Add remaining ingredients; mix well. Chill to blend flavors.

Yield: 12 servings. Leftovers will keep for several days in the refrigerator.

50 calories per serving, 0.3 g fat (0 g saturated), trace cholesterol, 2 g protein, 11 g carbohydrate, 225 mg sodium, 326 mg potassium, <1 mg iron, 3 g fiber, 60 mg calcium.

Variation:

- *Non-Dairy Version: Omit yogurt, mayonnaise and ketchup. Substitute 1½ cups bottled low-calorie Thousand Island salad dressing. If desired, fold in 1 cup of drained pineapple tidbits.*

Creamy Cucumber Salad

2 English cucumbers, thinly sliced
1 tsp salt
4 green onions, sliced
2 cloves garlic, crushed
1 cup non-fat yogurt or low-fat sour cream
2 tbsp vinegar
1 tbsp sugar
salt and pepper, to taste

1. Sprinkle cucumber slices with salt. Mix well; let stand for ½ hour. Press out excess liquid. Combine all ingredients in a bowl and mix gently, adding salt and pepper to taste. Serve chilled.

Yield: 6 servings. Leftovers will keep about a day in the refrigerator.

59 calories per serving, 0.2 g fat (0.1 g saturated), <1 mg cholesterol, 4 g protein, 12 g carbohydrate, 426 mg sodium, 276 mg potassium, <1 mg iron, 1 g fiber, 105 mg calcium.

Notes:
- *One clove of garlic contains 1 mg of calcium. If you eat 300 cloves, you'll get the same amount as in a glass of milk. You may have stronger bones, but you'll probably have less friends!*
- *Your processor can turn leftovers into Tzadziki in a flash. Process the mixture with quick on/offs, until desired texture is reached.*

Doug's "Flower Power" Caesar Salad

This super salad is nutrient-packed. It's a specialty of my son Doug, the Salad King!

3 cups broccoli flowerets
3 cups cauliflower flowerets
1 cup sliced red cabbage
3 tbsp grated Parmesan cheese
¾ cup Lighter Caesar Dressing (see page 105) or bottled low-fat Caesar dressing
½ tsp freshly ground pepper

1. Wash vegetables well; drain thoroughly. Combine all ingredients in a glass bowl and mix well. (Optional: Steam the veggies for 3 or 4 minutes if you prefer them softer.) This salad keeps for 3 days in a glass (not metal) bowl in the refrigerator, if well covered.

Yield: 6 servings.

68 calories per serving, 2.2 g fat (1.4 g saturated), 6 mg cholesterol, 6 g protein, 8 g carbohydrate, 401 mg sodium, 348 mg potassium, <1 mg iron, 3 g fiber, 148 mg calcium.

Easy Lentil Salad

2-19 oz (540 ml) cans lentils, rinsed and drained (or 4 cups cooked brown lentils)
2 cloves garlic, minced
1 red or yellow pepper, chopped
1 orange pepper, chopped
2 carrots, grated
6 green onions, chopped
¼ cup minced parsley
2 tbsp extra-virgin olive oil
3 tbsp lemon juice
salt and pepper, to taste
½ tsp each chili powder, dry mustard and cumin

1. Combine all ingredients in a large bowl and mix well. Season to taste. Cover and refrigerate.

Yield: 8 servings. This salad will keep in the refrigerator for up to 3 days if tightly covered.

173 calories per serving, 4.1 g fat (0.6 g saturated), 0 mg cholesterol, 10 g protein, 26 g carbohydrate, 247 mg sodium, 551 mg potassium, 4 mg iron, 9 g fiber, 41 mg calcium.

Variations:
- ***Kidney Bean and Chickpea Salad:*** *Instead of lentils, substitute 1 can of red kidney beans and 1 can of chickpeas, rinsed and drained.*
- ***Quick Couscous Salad:*** *Omit lentils; substitute 2 cups of couscous. Add 4 cups of water or chicken broth. Let stand for 10 minutes to absorb liquid. Add remaining ingredients; mix well.*

- *Instead of chili powder, dry mustard and cumin, add 3 to 4 tablespoons minced basil. Add ½ cup chopped roasted red peppers and ½ cup chopped sun-dried tomatoes to either version of the above salad.*

SALAD QUICKIES
- ***Quick Caesar Pasta Salad:*** Cook a 12-ounce package of bow tie pasta according to package directions. Drain and rinse well. Mix with ½ to ¾ cup Lighter Caesar Salad Dressing (see page 105) or bottled low-cal Caesar dressing. Add ½ cup each chopped red pepper, green onion and basil. Season to taste.
- ***New Potato Salad:*** Steam 2 pounds of new potatoes until tender-firm. When cool, cut in half but do not peel. Toss with ½ to ¾ cup low-cal vinaigrette dressing or Ranch-Style Dressing (see page 112). Add ½ cup each of minced celery and green onions. Season to taste.

Fattouche Salad

A fresh and lemony Middle-Eastern salad. Toasted pita is added just before serving. Yummy!

2 medium pitas
1 bunch flat-leaf or curly parsley
1 head iceberg or Romaine lettuce
2–3 ripe tomatoes, diced
½ of an English cucumber, diced
4 green onions (or 1 small onion, diced)

Dressing:
juice of 1 lemon (3 tbsp)
2 tbsp fresh mint, finely chopped
3–4 tbsp olive oil (preferably extra-virgin)
1 clove garlic, crushed (optional)
salt and pepper, to taste

1. Split pitas in half and place on an un-greased baking sheet. Bake in a preheated 400°F oven until crisp, about 10 minutes. Break pitas into small pieces and set aside. Wash parsley and lettuce; dry well. Mince parsley leaves; tear lettuce in bite-sized pieces. In a large bowl, combine lettuce, parsley, tomatoes, cucumber and onions; chill. Combine dressing ingredients; set aside. Just before serving, combine all ingredients and mix well. Serve immediately.

Yield: 6 servings. Leftover salad will become soggy.

150 calories per serving, 7.7 g fat (1.1 g saturated), 0 mg cholesterol, 4 g protein, 18 g carbohydrate, 127 mg sodium, 386 mg potassium, 2 mg iron, 3 g fiber, 62 mg calcium.

Fennel, Orange and Spinach Salad

Fennel, also known as finocchio, has a mild licorice flavor. The fronds (leaves) resemble fresh dill.

    1 medium bulb fennel (about ½ lb)
    ½ of a 10-oz pkg fresh spinach
    4 large seedless oranges
    1 red pepper, halved, seeded and thinly sliced
    ½ cup chopped red onion (or 4 green onions)
    2 tbsp lemon juice or rice vinegar
    1 clove garlic, crushed
    1 tsp honey-style mustard
    2 tbsp extra-virgin olive oil
    salt and pepper, to taste

1. Wash fennel; remove any stringy or brown outer stalks. Chop some of the fronds and reserve. Trim away root end. Slice fennel bulbs and stems into ¼-inch slices and place in a serving bowl. Trim away tough stems

99

from spinach. Wash spinach, dry well and tear into bite-size pieces. Peel oranges with a sharp knife, removing the white pith. Cut in half and slice thinly. Combine oranges in a bowl with fennel, spinach, red pepper and onion. Refrigerate until serving time. In a small bowl, combine lemon juice, garlic and mustard. Whisk in oil; refrigerate.

2. At serving time, pour dressing over fennel mixture and toss to coat with dressing. Season with salt and pepper. Garnish with fennel fronds.

Yield: 8 servings. So refreshing!

95 calories per serving, 3.7 g fat (0.5 g saturated), 0 mg cholesterol, 2 g protein, 16 g carbohydrate, 34 mg sodium, 398 mg potassium, <1 mg iron, 4 g fiber, 68 mg calcium.

Note:
- *To test fennel for freshness, press the flesh lightly with your thumb. Avoid any bulbs that are soft.*

Variation:
- **Turkey, Fennel and Orange Salad:** *Turn this salad into a main course by topping it with 2 cups of julienned smoked turkey (or chicken).*

Greek Salad

I've reduced the fat content considerably for this marvelous Mediterranean salad, but not the flavor! It's perfect for a buffet. Double or triple the recipe for a large crowd since it disappears so quickly.

4 firm, ripe tomatoes
3 green peppers (or 1 green, 1 red, 1 yellow)
1 English cucumber, peeled
½ of a red or Spanish onion (about 1 cup)
¼ cup pitted black olives
½ cup feta cheese, finely diced or grated

2 tbsp olive oil (preferably extra-virgin)
juice of a lemon (3 tbsp)
salt and pepper, to taste
½ tsp each dried basil and oregano

1. Cut tomatoes, peppers, cucumber and onion into 1-inch chunks. Slice olives or cut them in half. Combine all ingredients in a large bowl and toss to mix. (Can be prepared several hours in advance and refrigerated.)

Yield: 6 servings of about 1 cup each. Leftovers keep for 1 or 2 days in the refrigerator.

136 calories per serving, 8.5 g fat (2.7 g saturated), 11 mg cholesterol, 4 g protein, 13 g carbohydrate, 202 mg sodium, 473 mg potassium, 1 mg iron, 3 g fiber, 93 mg calcium.

Variation:
- ***Lactose-Free Greek Salad:*** *Substitute extra-firm tofu (preferably lite) for feta cheese. Slice tofu; place slices between 2 layers of paper towels. Cover with a baking sheet and top with several cans to press out excess liquid. Let stand 20 minutes. Dice tofu and add to salad. Add 2 to 3 tablespoons of Parmesan-flavored soy or rice cheese. Toss gently to mix.*

Greek-Style Black Bean Salad

So colorful, so good! Silken tofu can be substituted for the feta cheese for a non-dairy version.

2-19 oz (540 ml) cans black beans, rinsed and drained (or 4 cups cooked black beans)
¾ cup chopped red onion
1 yellow pepper, chopped
1 red pepper, chopped
2–3 tbsp extra-virgin olive oil
3 tbsp fresh lemon juice

¼ cup fresh mint leaves, minced
¼ cup fresh parsley leaves, minced
salt and freshly ground pepper, to taste
2 firm tomatoes, chopped
½ cup feta cheese, crumbled

1. Combine all ingredients except tomatoes and cheese; mix well. Marinate for at least 20 to 30 minutes. Adjust seasonings to taste and garnish with tomatoes and cheese just before serving.

Yield: 8 servings.

199 calories per serving, 6.9 g fat (1.9 g saturated), 8 mg cholesterol, 11 g protein, 26 g carbohydrate, 585 mg sodium, 185 mg potassium, 4 mg iron, 9 g fiber, 107 mg calcium.

Honey Mustard Carrot Salad

2 lb carrots, peeled and grated
4 green onions, chopped
2 tbsp chopped parsley and/or dill
3 tbsp honey
1 tbsp Dijon mustard (to taste)
1 tbsp extra-virgin olive oil
⅓ cup raisins, rinsed and drained
1 tbsp orange juice
1 tbsp lemon juice
salt and pepper, to taste

1. Combine all ingredients in a bowl and toss to mix. Adjust seasonings to taste. Serve chilled.

Yield: 6 servings.

115 calories per serving, 2.2 g fat (0.3 g saturated), 0 mg cholesterol, 2 g protein, 25 g carbohydrate, 90 mg sodium, 454 mg potassium, <1 mg iron, 4 g fiber, 43 mg calcium.

Honey Mustard Dressing

Fabulous! Use as a dressing over salad greens or as a sauce for poached salmon for rave reviews!

　　¼ cup olive oil (preferably extra-virgin)
　　¼ cup white or rice wine vinegar (or 2 tbsp orange juice and 2 tbsp vinegar)
　　⅓ cup liquid honey
　　2 tbsp Dijon or prepared mustard
　　¼ cup water
　　freshly ground pepper

1.　Combine all ingredients in a jar, cover and shake well. Keeps in the refrigerator for up to a month.

Yield: About 1 cup.

42 calories per tbsp, 2.7 g fat (0.4 g saturated), 0 mg cholesterol, trace protein, 5 g carbohydrate, 36 mg sodium, 9 mg potassium, trace iron, 0 g fiber, 2 mg calcium.

Israeli Salad

I love to cook, but don't always have the patience to chop vegetables into the small cubes that make this salad so delicious. Bring a small taste of Israel to your table! This is a favorite at a buffet. Recipe can be halved, if desired.

　　1 head of Romaine or iceberg lettuce
　　4 green onions
　　1 medium onion
　　2 green peppers

1 red pepper
1 English cucumber, peeled
8 firm, ripe tomatoes (preferably Israeli)
4 tbsp olive oil (preferably extra-virgin)
4 tbsp fresh lemon juice
1 tsp salt (or to taste)
freshly ground pepper, optional

1. Wash and dry vegetables well. Dice them neatly into ½-inch pieces and combine in a large bowl. Sprinkle with olive oil and lemon juice. Add seasonings; mix again. Adjust seasonings to taste.

Yield: 8 servings. Salad tastes best eaten the same day it is made, but leftovers will keep for a day in the refrigerator. Drain off excess liquid in the bottom of the bowl before serving.

127 calories per serving, 7.7 g fat (1.1 g saturated), 0 mg cholesterol, 3 g protein, 14 g carbohydrate, 600 mg sodium, 637 mg potassium, 2 mg iron, 4 g fiber, 45 mg calcium.

Variation:
- ***Mediterranean Vegetable Salad:*** *Add ½ cup sliced black olives, ½ cup sliced radishes and ½ cup chopped fresh parsley or coriander/cilantro.*

Jodi's Famous Bean Salad

My daughter Jodi is always asked to bring this terrific bean salad to dinner parties and barbecues. Thank goodness it's so easy to make. My granddaughter Lauren just loves it!

19 oz (540 ml) can black beans
19 oz (540 ml) can chickpeas
19 oz (540 ml) can lentils

2 cloves garlic, crushed
1 green and/or red pepper, chopped
1 yellow pepper, chopped
½ cup red onion, chopped
¼ cup coriander/cilantro, minced
¼ cup extra-virgin olive oil
¼ cup balsamic vinegar
1 tsp ground cumin (or to taste)
salt and freshly ground black pepper

1. Rinse beans, chickpeas and lentils; drain well. Combine all ingredients in a large mixing bowl; mix well. Season to taste. Cover and refrigerate. This tastes even better the next day!

Yield: 12 servings. This salad will keep for up to 3 days in the refrigerator if tightly covered.

172 calories per serving, 6.1 g fat (0.7 g saturated), 0 mg cholesterol, 8 g protein, 23 g carbohydrate, 238 mg sodium, 190 mg potassium, 3 mg iron, 8 g fiber, 41 mg calcium.

Lighter Caesar Salad Dressing
Creamy and delicious. You won't miss the fat!

½ cup non-fat yogurt
¼ cup fat-free or low-fat mayonnaise
1 clove garlic, crushed
¼ cup grated Parmesan cheese
½ tsp Worcestershire sauce
2 tbsp lemon juice (to taste)
¾ tsp salt (to taste)
freshly ground pepper, to taste

1.   Combine all ingredients and mix well; chill. Delicious over Romaine
      lettuce or spinach.

Yield: about 1 cup. Dressing will keep 4 or 5 days in the refrigerator.

*15 calories per tbsp, 0.6 g fat (0.4 g saturated), 2 mg cholesterol, 1 g protein,
2 g carbohydrate, 168 mg sodium, 27 mg potassium, 0 mg iron, 0 g fiber, 37 mg
calcium.*

Orange Balsamic Vinaigrette

Wonderful on mixed salad greens. It also makes a yummy marinade for
boneless chicken breasts.

   ¼ cup olive or canola oil
   6 tbsp orange juice
   ¼ cup balsamic vinegar
   1–2 cloves garlic, crushed
   2 tbsp minced fresh basil (or ½ tsp dried)
   1 tbsp sugar salt and pepper, to taste

1.   Combine all ingredients and mix well. Dressing will keep in the
      refrigerator about 2 weeks.

Yield: About ¾ cup.

*43 calories per tbsp, 3.7 g fat (0.5 g saturated), 0 mg cholesterol, trace protein, 2 g
carbohydrate, 1 mg sodium, 15 mg potassium, trace iron, 0 g fiber, 2 mg calcium.*

Oriental Cole Slaw

Sesame oil and rice vinegar enhance the flavor of this non-traditional cole slaw. Addictive!

> 1 medium head green cabbage (8 cup shredded)
> 2–3 carrots, grated
> ¾ cup thinly sliced red onion (or 6 green onions, sliced)
> 2–3 cloves garlic, crushed
> ⅓ cup canola oil
> ⅓ cup rice vinegar
> ¼ cup sugar
> 2 tsp Oriental sesame oil
> salt and pepper, to taste

1. Combine cabbage, carrots, onions and garlic in a large mixing bowl. Combine canola oil and rice vinegar with sugar in a 2-cup Pyrex measure. Microwave uncovered on HIGH for 45 seconds, until almost boiling. Pour hot dressing over cabbage mixture. Add sesame oil and mix well. Season to taste.

Yield: 12 servings. Leftovers will keep about a week in the refrigerator.

98 calories per serving, 7 g fat (0.6 g saturated), 0 mg cholesterol, <1 g protein, 9 g carbohydrate, 13 mg sodium, 171 mg potassium, trace iron, 2 g fiber, 28 mg calcium.

Oriental Cucumber Salad

> 2 English cucumbers (unpeeled), thinly sliced
> ½ of a small red onion, thinly sliced
> 1 red pepper, thinly sliced
> 1 tsp minced ginger
> ¼ cup rice vinegar

2 tsp Oriental sesame oil
1 tbsp sugar
1 tsp salt (or to taste)
½ tsp pepper

1. Combine all ingredients in a bowl and mix well. Adjust seasonings to taste.

Yield: 6 servings. Leftovers will keep for a day in the refrigerator.

30 calories per serving, 0.2 g fat (0 g saturated), 0 mg cholesterol, 1 g protein, 7 g carbohydrate, 391 mg sodium, 191 mg potassium, trace iron, 1 g fiber, 19 mg calcium.

Variations:
*   *Add 2 tablespoons orange juice and 1 teaspoon soy sauce.*
*   ***Old-Fashioned Cucumber Salad:*** *Omit ginger and sesame oil. Use white vinegar instead of rice vinegar and increase sugar to 2 tablespoons. Use Spanish onion instead of red onion, if desired.*

Note:
*   *The liquid at the bottom of the bowl can be used as a yummy guilt-free dressing over salad greens!*

Pesto Pasta Salad

Excellent for a summer salad buffet, and so pretty. If you don't have pesto on hand, add 2 cloves of freshly crushed garlic and 3 tablespoons grated Parmesan cheese.

12-oz pkg (340 g) spiral pasta or 3-color rotini
2 cups frozen mixed vegetables (e.g., broccoli, cauliflower and carrots)
6 green onions, chopped

2 green peppers, chopped
1 red pepper, chopped
¼ cup parsley, minced
¼ cup fresh basil leaves, minced
3 tbsp Best-O Pesto (see page 149), to taste
3 tbsp extra-virgin olive oil
2 tbsp lemon juice
⅓–½ cup non-fat yogurt or mayonnaise
salt and pepper, to taste

1. Cook pasta according to package directions. Drain well. Cook vegetables according to package directions. Let cool. In a large bowl, combine all ingredients and mix well. Adjust seasonings to taste. Chill at least 2 or 3 hours or overnight to allow flavors to blend.

Yield: 10 servings. Leftovers will keep for 2 or 3 days in the refrigerator. Do not freeze.

209 calories per serving, 5.7 g fat (0.8 g saturated), trace cholesterol, 7 g protein, 34 g carbohydrate, 35 mg sodium, 256 mg potassium, 2 mg iron, 4 fiber, 59 mg calcium.

Variations:

- *Substitute bow-tie pasta for 3-color pasta. As a vegetarian main dish, add 1 to 2 cups canned chickpeas, rinsed and drained. If needed, add a little extra yogurt or mayonnaise to moisten.*
- ***Pareve* Pasta Salad:** Use low-fat mayo instead of yogurt. Omit Pesto; add 1 teaspoon Dijon mustard. *Pareve means dairy-free.*
- ***Salmon Pasta Salad:** Add 2 cups of cooked canned salmon, in chunks. Dill can replace basil.*

Quinoa Mandarin Salad

For extra crunch, garnish with toasted sesame seeds. The processor will help you prepare this salad quickly. Quinoa is also great in tabbouleh.

3 cups cooked, cooled quinoa
½ cup minced parsley
2 tbsp minced fresh basil
2 slices of ginger, minced (1 tbsp)
2 green onions, minced
½ of a red pepper, diced
10-oz can mandarin oranges, drained
1 cup snow peas, trimmed and cut in ½" strips
2 tbsp soy or tamari sauce
2 tbsp rice vinegar
1 tbsp Oriental sesame oil
salt and pepper, to taste

1. Cook quinoa as directed; cool completely. Combine quinoa with remaining ingredients and mix gently. Adjust seasonings to taste. Chill before serving.

Yield: 6 servings. Leftovers will keep about 2 days in the refrigerator. Do not freeze.

160 calories per serving, 4.2 g fat (0.7 g saturated), 0 mg cholesterol, 5 g protein, 27 g carbohydrate, 368 mg sodium, 369 mg potassium, 4 mg iron, 3 g fiber, 40 mg calcium.

Rainbow Tabbouleh Salad

This colorful, vitamin-packed salad is guaranteed to be a winner on any buffet table! It's also a wonderful way to use up fresh mint if you grow it in your garden.

⅓ cup bulgur or couscous
⅔ cup boiling water
2 cups minced flat-leaf or curly parsley
1 cup mint leaves
1 green and 1 red pepper
4 firm, ripe tomatoes
4 green onions (scallions)
¼ cup red onion
¼ cup grated carrots
½ of an English cucumber, seeded and diced
¼–⅓ cup olive oil (to taste)
¼–⅓ cup fresh lemon juice (to taste)
salt and pepper, to taste
1 tbsp fresh basil, chopped (or 1 tsp dried)
fresh mint or basil leaves, to garnish

1. In a small bowl, combine bulgur or couscous with boiling water. Let stand for 20 minutes to soften. (Couscous will take only 10 minutes.) Meanwhile, soak parsley and mint in cold salted water for 15 to 20 minutes. Drain and dry well. Trim off tough parsley stems. Remove mint leaves from stems.

2. Mince parsley and mint leaves. Chop vegetables. (Do this in the processor in batches, using on/off turns to retain texture.) Combine parsley, mint and vegetables in a large mixing bowl. Add drained bulgur or couscous, olive oil and lemon juice. Mix well. Add salt, pepper and basil. Allow to stand for at least ½ hour for flavors to blend. Garnish with fresh mint or basil leaves.

Yield: 8 servings. Leftovers will keep for 2 or 3 days in the refrigerator.

121 calories per serving, 7.4 g fat (1 g saturated), 0 mg cholesterol, 3 g protein, 14 g carbohydrate, 22 mg sodium, 434 mg potassium, 2 mg iron, 4 g fiber, 47 mg calcium.

Notes:
- *Store bulgur in an airtight container in a cool, dark place. It can be stored in the refrigerator for several months, or in the freezer for up to a year.*
- *Reserve parsley stems and use them when making chicken or vegetable broth.*
- *Parsley should be well dried before chopping. Your processor makes quick work of this task. Measure parsley after chopping. You need approximately twice as much before chopping to give you the required amount for this recipe.*
- *If fresh mint is not available, add 2 teaspoons dried mint. If you don't have dried mint, just leave it out. The salad will still have a delicious, garden-fresh flavor.*

Variations:
- *Increase bulgur or couscous to 1 cup for a grain-based Tabbouleh. Soak the grain in double the amount of water.*
- ***Traditional Tabbouleh:*** *Omit red onion, carrots, cucumber and basil.*
- ***Quinoa Tabbouleh:*** *Use 1 cup of cooked quinoa instead of soaked bulgur or couscous.*
- ***Greek-Style Tabbouleh:*** *Crumble or grate ½ cup feta cheese over Tabbouleh. Add ⅓ cup sliced black olives. One serving contains 152 calories, 10 g fat (2.5 g saturated) and 98 mg calcium.*

Ranch-Style Dressing

¾ cup non-fat yogurt
¼ cup fat-free mayonnaise
1 tbsp white or cider vinegar

½ tsp sugar
2 tsp Dijon mustard
1 green onion, finely minced
1 clove garlic, crushed
¼ tsp dried thyme
freshly ground pepper

1. Measure all ingredients into a small bowl. Mix well and refrigerate. Serve chilled. Stir before using.

Yield: About 1 cup. Dressing will keep about 4 or 5 days in the refrigerator.

9 calories per tbsp 0.1 g fat (0 g saturated), trace cholesterol, <1 g protein, 1 g carbohydrate, 42 mg sodium, 29 mg potassium, trace iron, 0 g fiber, 21 mg calcium.

Red Cabbage Cole Slaw

The boiled dressing transforms the cabbage into a beautiful, brilliant magenta color.

1 medium red cabbage, cored and thinly sliced (about 8 cups)
4 green onions, thinly sliced
1 medium carrot, grated
2 tbsp canola oil
¼ cup red or white wine vinegar (also excellent with raspberry or balsamic vinegar)
2 tbsp sugar
salt and pepper, to taste

1. Combine vegetables in a large mixing bowl. In a medium saucepan, combine oil, vinegar and sugar. Bring to a boil. (Or combine in a 2-cup Pyrex measure and microwave uncovered for 45 seconds.) Pour hot dressing over vegetables. Mix well. Add salt and pepper to taste. Refrigerate to blend flavors.

Yield: 12 servings. Leftovers keep 3 to 4 days in the refrigerator.

45 calories per serving, 2.4 g fat (0.2 g saturated), 0 mg cholesterol, <1 g protein, 6 g carbohydrate, 8 mg sodium, 132 mg potassium, trace iron, 1 g fiber, 28 mg calcium.

Shake It Up Salad Dressing

You'll twist and shout about this salad dressing. It contains less than a gram of fat per tablespoon! So simple, so guilt-free. It can also be used as a marinade for chicken or fish.

¾ cup tomato or vegetable juice
3 tbsp balsamic or red wine vinegar
1 tbsp olive oil (preferably extra-virgin)
1–2 cloves garlic, crushed
1 tsp sugar (to taste)
½ tsp Worcestershire sauce (to taste)
½ tsp dry mustard
½ tsp dried basil

1. Measure all ingredients into a jar. Cover and shake well to blend. Refrigerate dressing. Shake well before serving. Serve over your favorite greens.

Yield: About 1 cup. Dressing keeps for 2 or 3 weeks in the refrigerator.

14 calories per tbsp, 0.9 g fat (0.1 g saturated), 0 mg cholesterol, trace protein, 1 g carbohydrate, 41 mg sodium, 27 mg potassium, trace iron, trace fiber, 3 mg calcium.

Simply Basic Vinaigrette
A light and luscious vinaigrette salad dressing.

¼ cup olive or canola oil
¼ cup rice, balsamic or red wine vinegar
¼ cup chicken or vegetable broth
1 tsp Dijon mustard
1 tbsp honey or maple syrup
½ tsp dried basil (or 1 tbsp fresh minced)
1 clove garlic, crushed
salt and freshly ground pepper, to taste

1.   Combine all ingredients and mix well. Drizzle over your favorite salad greens and toss to mix.

Yield: about ¾ cup dressing. Leftovers can be refrigerated for 2 or 3 days.

43 calories per tbsp, 4.1 g fat (0.6 g saturated), 0 mg cholesterol, trace protein, 1 g carbohydrate, 12 mg sodium, 4 mg potassium, trace iron, 0 g fiber, 3 mg calcium.

Variations:
- ***Orange Vinaigrette:*** *Use ¼ cup of orange juice instead of chicken or vegetable broth. Dressing will keep for 2 weeks.*
- ***Poppy Seed Dressing:*** *Combine ¼ cup canola oil, ¼ cup rice vinegar, 2 tablespoons orange juice, 2 tablespoons lemon juice and ¼ cup sugar in a saucepan. Bring to a boil. Add 1 teaspoon poppy seeds, ¾ teaspoon Dijon mustard and a dash of salt. When cool, store in a jar in the refrigerator. Shake well to blend before serving. One tablespoon of dressing contains 47 calories, 3.7 grams fat (0.2 grams saturated) and 4 grams carbohydrate.*

Note:
- *If dressing is refrigerated, olive oil will congeal. Just let dressing stand at room temperature for a few minutes before serving; shake well.*

Spinach and Mushroom Salad with Honey Mustard Dressing

10-oz pkg (300 g) fresh spinach
½ cup mushrooms, thinly sliced
½ of a red onion, thinly sliced (about ½ cup)
1 small carrot, grated
½ cup Honey Mustard Dressing (see page 103)

1. Trim tough stems from spinach leaves. Wash and dry thoroughly; tear into bite-size pieces. Combine all vegetables in a large bowl. Prepare salad dressing and set aside. (Vegetables and dressing can be prepared in advance and refrigerated separately for several hours.) At serving time, combine all ingredients and toss gently to mix. Serve immediately.

Yield: 6 servings. Leftover salad will become soggy.

91 calories per serving, 4.9 g fat (0.7 g saturated), 0 mg cholesterol, 2 g protein, 12 g carbohydrate, 95 mg sodium, 289 mg potassium, 1 mg iron, 2 g fiber, 43 mg calcium.

Notes:
- *Fresh spinach can be very sandy and gritty. Immerse trimmed spinach leaves in a sink full of cold water. Swish the leaves around and then let stand for a few minutes. Lift spinach from water, leaving sand and dirt behind in the bottom of the sink. Repeat until water is clean. Dry spinach thoroughly (in a salad spinner or by wrapping in a clean towel). Wrap spinach in paper towels and place in a sealed plastic storage bag. Refrigerate for up to 4 days.*
- *Time-Saving Tip: Washed baby spinach greens can be used instead of regular spinach. This saves time and clean up!*

116

- *Did you know that spinach isn't an especially good source of calcium or iron? It contains oxalates, which reduce absorption of calcium, iron and other minerals.*

Variation:

- ***Spinach, Mandarin and Almond Salad:*** *Omit mushrooms. Use 2 tablespoons rice vinegar and 2 tablespoons orange juice in the salad dressing. Combine spinach, onion and grated carrot in a bowl. Add ¾ cup canned mandarin oranges, drained and patted dry. You can also add ½ cup bean sprouts. Add dressing; toss gently to mix. Garnish with ¼ cup toasted slivered almonds or pine nuts.*

Strawberries with Balsamic Vinegar or Red Wine

See recipe under Desserts, in chapter 7, page 259.

Thousand Island Dressing (or Dip)

½ cup non-fat yogurt
½ cup non-fat or low-fat mayonnaise
⅓ cup chili sauce or ketchup
3 tbsp relish
2 tbsp minced onion
1 tsp lemon juice (to taste)
salt and pepper, to taste

1. Combine all ingredients and mix well. Cover and refrigerate.

Yield: About 1½ cups. Dressing will keep 4 or 5 days in the refrigerator.

11 calories per tbsp 0 g fat (0 g saturated), trace cholesterol, trace protein, 2 g carbohydrate, 92 mg sodium, 27 mg potassium, 0 mg iron, trace fiber, 10 mg calcium.

Tofu Antipasto

Debbie Jeremias likes to serve this as one of several salads for special occasions. It goes like crazy!

 1 cup mushrooms, quartered
 2 stalks celery, sliced
 3 medium ripe tomatoes, diced
 1 red pepper, diced
 1 yellow pepper, diced
 1 orange pepper, diced
 2 green onions, sliced
 2 cloves garlic, thinly sliced
 ⅓–½ cup pitted black olives, halved
 ¾ lb firm tofu, diced (about 1½ cups)
 2 tbsp balsamic vinegar
 2 tbsp olive oil (preferably extra-virgin)
 1 tsp dried oregano
 1 tsp dried basil
 sea salt and freshly ground pepper, to taste

1. Combine all ingredients in a large bowl and mix well. If you have time, let mixture stand for 20 to 30 minutes to develop the flavor. (Can be made several hours in advance and refrigerated.)

Yield: 8 servings. Leftovers will keep for 2 or 3 days in the refrigerator.

140 calories per serving, 8.2 g fat (1.2 g saturated), 0 mg cholesterol, 8 g protein, 12 g carbohydrate, 73 mg sodium, 454 mg potassium, 6 mg iron, 3 g fiber, 116 mg calcium.

Note:

- *To lower calories and fat, use 1% silken extra-firm tofu. A 3-ounce (84 g) serving of tofu contains 35 calories and 1 g fat. Its texture is softer than regular firm tofu, but it works well in this recipe.*

Tomato, Onion and Pepper Salad

3–4 firm, ripe tomatoes, in 8ths
1 cup thinly sliced Spanish or red onions
½ of a red pepper, sliced
½ of a green pepper, sliced
½ of a yellow pepper, sliced
2 tbsp fresh basil, chopped (or 1 tsp dried)
2 cloves garlic, crushed
2 tbsp olive oil (preferably extra-virgin)
2 tbsp fresh lemon juice or balsamic vinegar
salt and freshly ground pepper
½ tsp Dijon mustard, optional

1. Combine tomatoes, onions, peppers, basil and garlic in a large bowl. (Can be prepared a few hours in advance, covered and refrigerated.) Add remaining ingredients and toss gently. Serve immediately.

Yield: 6 servings. Leftovers will keep about a day in the refrigerator.

72 calories per serving, 4.9 g fat (0.7 g saturated), 0 mg cholesterol, 1 g protein, 7 g carbohydrate, 9 mg sodium, 281 mg potassium, <1 mg iron, 2 g fiber, 12 mg calcium.

THE PERFECT DAYTIME LOW GI BEVERAGE

Florida Water à la Doris

Similar to Cover Photo! Doris Fink, my Montreal assistant, always prepared a pitcher of this refreshing water for my students! This citrus water can help to lower the GI content of your meals when you drink it with them. It's also perfect anytime of day.

1.   Place 2 sliced oranges, 2 sliced lemons and/or limes in a large pitcher. Fill with ice-cold water (preferably spring water). Serve chilled. Simply refreshing! (Contains no calories.)

■ SANDWICHES, FILLINGS AND SPREADS

All of the following recipes are intended for low GI breads (see chapter 1, page 25 and chapter 4, under Breads).

Best Cottage Cheese

(See recipe, page 46.)

Better than Butter Spread

(See recipe, page 63.)

Chickpea Mock Chopped Liver

Canned lentils can be substituted for chickpeas.

   3 medium onions
   1½ cups cooked or canned chickpeas, rinsed and drained
   2 tbsp almonds or walnuts, optional
   2 hard-boiled eggs (or 1 hard-boiled egg plus 2 hard-boiled whites)
   salt and pepper, to taste
   1 tsp honey

1. Preheat oven to 400°F. Place unpeeled onions on a baking sheet and bake for 40 minutes, until soft. (Or pierce onions in 3 or 4 places with a sharp knife; place on a plate and microwave on HIGH for 6 to 8 minutes.) Cool slightly; remove peel. Combine all ingredients in processor. Process 30 seconds, until finely chopped. If mixture seems dry, blend in a little water. Chill before serving.

Yield: About 2¾ cups. Mixture keeps for 3 or 4 days in the refrigerator. It can be frozen, but season mixture lightly because the pepper's flavor will become stronger.

74 calories per ¼ cup, 2.4 g fat (0.4 g saturated), 39 mg cholesterol, 4 g protein, 10 g carbohydrate, 14 mg sodium, 132 mg potassium, <1 mg iron, 2 g fiber, 25 mg calcium.

Creamy Salmon Paté (Mock Salmon Mousse)

This easy, tasty spread is a good source of calcium, but be sure to add the mashed salmon bones.

4 green onions, minced
2 tbsp fresh dill, minced
½ lb (250 g) smooth cottage cheese or low-fat cream cheese
¼ cup non-fat yogurt or sour cream
7½ oz can (213 g) salmon, drained
1 tsp lemon juice (preferably fresh)
freshly ground pepper

1. Combine all ingredients and mix until blended. (If using the processor, first mince green onions and dill, then add remaining ingredients and process just until blended.) Chill before serving. Serve as a spread with low GI crackers, breads or fresh veggies, or use as a sandwich filling. If desired, garnish with finely minced red onion, thinly sliced cucumber and/or dill.

Yield: About 1½ cups. Mixture will keep about 3 days in the refrigerator. Do not freeze.

55 calories per ¼ cup, 1.6 g fat (0.4 g saturated), 11 mg cholesterol, 8 g protein, 2 g carbohydrate, 197 mg sodium, 128 mg potassium, trace iron, trace fiber, 80 mg calcium.

Variations:
- **Smoked Salmon Paté:** *Add 1 teaspoon liquid smoke and 1 teaspoon Worcestershire sauce.*
- **Tuna Paté:** *Instead of salmon, use water-packed tuna in the above recipe.*

Dijon Mustard Sauce
Delicious with fish, or use as a zesty spread for your favorite sandwich.

2 tbsp Dijon mustard
2 tbsp fat-free or light mayonnaise
1 clove garlic, crushed
¼ tsp Worcestershire sauce
3–4 drops of lemon juice

1. Combine all ingredients and mix to blend.

Yield: About ¼ cup. Serve chilled. Do not freeze.

14 calories per tbsp, 0.6 g fat (0 g saturated), 0 mg cholesterol, <1 g protein, 2 g carbohydrate, 216 mg sodium, 20 mg potassium, trace iron, trace fiber, 11 mg calcium.

Good for You Kangaroo Pita Pockets!
Minis make great appetizers; regular-sized pitas make a healthy lunch box choice!

  6 medium pitas or 24 mini pitas
  1 cup Healthier Hummus (see page 278)
  ½ cup chopped red pepper
  ½ cup chopped green pepper
  3 tomatoes, cored, halved and thinly sliced
  ½ cup thinly sliced Spanish or red onion
  1 English cucumber, thinly sliced
  ½ cup alfalfa sprouts

1.   Cut medium-size pitas in half to make 12 pockets (or slit mini pitas open along one edge). Spread insides with Hummous. Fill with peppers, tomatoes, onions, cucumbers; top with sprouts.

Yield: 12 medium pockets or 24 minis. One medium or 2 minis make 1 serving. Do not freeze.

135 calories per serving, 2.2 g fat (0.3 g saturated), 0 mg cholesterol, 5 g protein, 25 g carbohydrate, 166 mg sodium, 227 mg potassium, 2 mg iron, 2 g fiber, 44 mg calcium.

Notes and Variations:
- *Use miniature pitas for hors d'oeuvres. Fill with your favorite filling. Top with salsa, sliced onions, roasted red peppers, chutney, etc.*
- *Fill pita pockets with any of the vegetarian variations of Mock Chopped Liver (see pages 120 and 128).*
- *Lighter Chicken or Turkey Salad (see pages 142 and 144) are a nice change from chicken or tuna fillings.*
- *Thinly sliced roast turkey or chicken breast (homemade or deli-style) make easy, tasty fillings. Mix fat-free mayonnaise with Dijon or honey-style mustard to moisten the inside of pitas.*

- *Stir-fry vegetables make an excellent filling for pita pockets. Add strips of chicken, turkey or tofu.*

Lighter Chicken Salad

(See further under Chicken and Turkey, pages 142 and 144.)

Lighter Chopped Egg Salad

Boil a few extra eggs and throw away half of the yolks. Limit your intake of egg yolks to 4 per week.

4 hard-boiled eggs
3 tbsp fat-free or light mayonnaise
1 stalk celery, minced
2 green onions, minced
1 tbsp minced dill, optional
salt and pepper, to taste

1. Cut cooked eggs in half and discard 2 of the yolks (or feed them to your dog). Mash remaining eggs. Mix with remaining ingredients and season to taste.

Yield: About 1 cup. Do not freeze.

49 calories per ¼ cup, 2.2 g fat (0.7 g saturated), 91 mg cholesterol, 4 g protein, 2 g carbohydrate, 181 mg sodium, 90 mg potassium, trace iron, trace fiber, 19 mg calcium.

Lighter Tuna Salad

Half a cup of tuna salad made with regular mayo contains nearly 200 calories and almost 10 grams of fat! Try it my way, with minced veggies added for crunch and fiber. You won't miss the fat!

6 ½ oz can (184 g) water-packed tuna
3–4 tbsp fat-free or light mayonnaise
1 stalk celery, finely chopped
2 green onions, minced (or ¼ cup red onion)
¼ cup finely grated carrot
1 tbsp dill or basil, minced (or ½ tsp dried)
freshly ground pepper, to taste
1 tbsp fresh lemon juice

1. Drain tuna thoroughly. Combine all ingredients and mix well. (The processor can be used to mince the vegetables. Add tuna and mayonnaise and process with quick on/offs, just until mixed. Do not over-process.) Use as a sandwich filling or serve as a spread with crackers. Alternately, serve a scoop of tuna salad on a bed of salad greens.

Yield: About 1¼ cups. Do not freeze.

48 calories per ¼ cup, 0.3 g fat (0.1 g saturated), 10 mg cholesterol, 8 g protein, 2 g carbohydrate, 172 mg sodium, 132 mg potassium, <1 mg iron, trace fiber, 11 mg calcium.

Variations:

- *Substitute 2 tablespoons non-fat yogurt for half the mayonnaise. Add ¼ cup minced red pepper and 1 teaspoon Dijon mustard. Parsley can replace dill or basil; ¼ cup minced radishes add great texture.*
- *Add 1 hard-boiled egg plus 2 hard-boiled egg whites to tuna mixture for a tasty mixture.*
- *Omit dill or basil. Add half of an 8-ounce can of water chestnuts, well-drained and finely minced, to tuna mixture. Add 1 teaspoon soy sauce and ½ teaspoon curry powder.*

Lighter Turkey Salad
(See further under Chicken and Turkey, pages 142 and 144.)

Mock Seafood Salad

1 lb (500 g) imitation crab (pollock), flaked
4 green onions, chopped
2 stalks celery, chopped
½ of a red or green pepper, chopped
2 tbsp fresh dill, minced (or 1 tsp dried)
3 tbsp fat-free or light mayonnaise
3 tbsp non-fat yogurt
1 tbsp fresh lemon juice
freshly ground pepper

1.   Combine ingredients and mix well. Serve chilled.

Yield: about 3 cups. Do not freeze. Leftovers will keep for a day or two in the refrigerator.

46 calories per ¼ cup, 0.5 g fat (0.1 g saturated), 8 mg cholesterol, 5 g protein, 5 g carbohydrate, 348 mg sodium, 82 mg potassium, trace iron, trace fiber, 19 mg calcium.

Notes:
- *As a main course, serve a generous scoop on a bed of salad greens. Top with sliced tomatoes, red onions and cucumbers. Garnish with thinly sliced lemon. To round out your meal (but not your hips), start out with a hearty bowl of Greek-Style Lentil Soup (see page 84)*
- *This mixture makes a nice stuffing for cherry tomatoes or mini pitas for your next party! It's also delicious as a sandwich filling with low GI breads.*

Molly Naimer's Green Pea Mock Liver

Molly Naimer lived at Manoir Montefiore, a Montreal senior residence where I was the food consultant. If you make her recipe, perhaps you'll also live into your nineties. When I asked Molly if this dish could be frozen, she replied "I don't know. I never had leftovers. It was always eaten up!"

1 large onion, finely diced
1 tbsp canola oil (approximately)
19 oz (540 ml) can green peas, drained and mashed
4 hard-boiled eggs, peeled and grated
8 walnut halves, chopped (not ground!)
salt and pepper, to taste

1.   In a non-stick skillet, brown onion in oil until crispy. Combine with remaining ingredients and mix well. Season to taste. Refrigerate to blend flavors. Use as a vegetarian alternative to chopped liver.

Yield: About 3 cups. Mixture keeps for 3 or 4 days in the fridge.

71 calories per ¼ cup, 4 g fat (0.7 g saturated), 73 mg cholesterol, 4 g protein, 5 g carbohydrate, 95 mg sodium, 98 mg potassium, <1 mg iron, 1 g fiber, 18 mg calcium.

Notes:
*   *If you discard 2 of the yolks, ¼ cup of the above spread will contain 64 calories, 38 milligrams cholesterol and 3.2 grams fat (0.5 grams saturated).*
*   *Compare the difference! An equal amount of chopped chicken livers with egg and onion has 132 calories, 212 milligrams cholesterol and 10.4 grams fat (3.2 grams saturated).*

Mushroom Mock Chopped Liver

Most recipes for mock liver are based on beans, peas or lentils. Sylvia Pleet of
Ottawa gave me this gem. I reduced the fat slightly to lighten it up.

2 tsp soft tub margarine or oil
2 large onions, sliced
2–3 tbsp water or vegetable broth
1 pint mushrooms, sliced
2 hard-boiled eggs (or 1 hard-boiled egg plus 2 hard-boiled whites)
2 tbsp finely chopped walnuts or almonds
Salt and pepper, to taste

1. Melt margarine in a skillet over medium heat. Add onions and sauté until
    nicely browned, about 5 minutes. If onions begin to stick, add water or
    broth as needed. Add mushrooms and sauté until well browned. When
    cool, combine with remaining ingredients in the processor. Process with
    quick on/offs.

Yield: About 2 cups. Serve chilled. Do not freeze.

*49 calories per ¼ cup, 2.8 g fat (0.5 g saturated), 40 mg cholesterol, 2 g protein, 5
g carbohydrate, 19 mg sodium, 129 mg potassium, <1 mg iron, <1 g fiber, 14 mg
calcium.*

- *Microwave Magic! Break 2 eggs into individual custard cups (or break 1 egg
  into a custard cup and the egg whites into another cup). Pierce yolk(s) with a
  fork to make an "X" (it doesn't matter if the yolks run). Cut 2 pieces of
  parchment paper and place them under running water. You'll then be able
  to mold the parchment paper around the custard cups! Microwave covered
  on MEDIUM (50%) for 2 to 2½ minutes, until firm. Let stand 1 minute.
  How "egg-citing"—hard-boiled eggs!*

Red Lentil Paté (I Can't Believe It's Not Chopped Liver!)

Savor the flavor of "almost-liver" without guilt or cholesterol. Thank you, Suzi Lipes.

2 cups red lentils, picked over and rinsed

4 cups vegetable broth or water

1 tbsp olive oil

2 large onions, chopped

3–4 cloves garlic, minced

1 tsp each dried basil, oregano and thyme

½ cup fresh parsley, minced

¼ cup seasoned breadcrumbs from low GI breads only (plus 2 tbsp to coat the pan)

½ tsp Kosher or sea salt (to taste)

freshly ground pepper (to taste)

2 tsp fresh lemon juice or balsamic vinegar

1 tsp Oriental sesame oil

1. Cook lentils in broth or water until tender, about 25 minutes. Do not drain. Let cool, then mash. Heat oil in a large non-stick skillet. Add onions, garlic and dried herbs. Sauté on medium heat until brown, stirring often. Add to lentils along with remaining ingredients; mix well. Preheat oven to 350°F. Spray a 9 x 4-inch loaf pan with non-stick spray. Sprinkle pan with 2 tablespoons crumbs, lightly coating bottom and sides of pan. Spread lentil mixture in pan. Bake uncovered for 30 minutes, until set. When cool, un-mold and refrigerate. Best served at room temperature.

Yield: 12 slices. Leftovers keep 3 to 4 days in the fridge. Freezing intensifies the flavor of the herbs.

144 calories per slice, 2.4 g fat (0.3 g saturated), trace cholesterol, 9 g protein, 23 g carbohydrate, 534 mg sodium, 379 mg potassium, 3 mg iron, 9 g fiber, 36 mg calcium.

Tofu Spread (Mock Egg Salad)

Don't tell them it's tofu! This tasty spread has fooled many guests who insist they detest tofu.

> 1 stalk celery
> 2 green onions
> 1 small carrot (about ¼ cup grated)
> 1 tbsp fresh dill and/or parsley, optional
> ½ lb (250 g) tofu
> 3 tbsp fat-free or light mayonnaise
> salt and pepper, to taste
> 2 tsp Dijon mustard

1. Mince vegetables very fine. Mash tofu. Combine all ingredients and mix until blended. (Can be done in the processor.) Chill. Serve with low GI crackers or breads, or use as a sandwich filling.

Yield: About 1¼ cups. Mixture will keep in the refrigerator for 2 or 3 days. Do not freeze.

63 calories per ¼ cup, 3.3 g fat (0.5 g saturated), 0 mg cholesterol, 6 g protein, 4 g carbohydrate, 103 mg sodium, 134 mg potassium, 4 mg iron, 1 g fiber, 83 mg calcium.

Notes:
- *Different brands of tofu vary in moisture content, so you may need a bit more mayonnaise to hold the mixture together.*
- *Non-fat yogurt can replace part of the mayonnaise, if desired.*

Vegetarian Harvest Roll-Ups (Fajitas)
Wrap it up! So colorful, so healthy.

2 cups eggplant, unpeeled, cut into strips
1 red and 1 yellow pepper, cut into strips
1 red onion, halved and cut into strips
1 zucchini, unpeeled, cut into strips
2 cups sliced mushrooms
3–4 cloves garlic, crushed
1 tbsp olive oil
2 tbsp balsamic vinegar or lemon juice
salt and pepper, to taste
2 tbsp minced fresh basil (or 2 tsp dried)
3 soft flour tortillas or very thin pitas (preferably whole wheat)
½ cup grated low-fat Mozzarella cheese, if desired

1. Either preheat broiler, or preheat oven to 425°F. Mix all ingredients together in a large bowl. (May be prepared in advance up to this point, covered and refrigerated for 3 or 4 hours.) Spread in a thin layer on a sprayed foil-lined baking sheet. Place pan on top rack of oven. Either broil for 10 to 12 minutes, or bake uncovered for 25 to 30 minutes, until tender-crisp and golden, stirring once or twice.
2. Spread hot vegetables in a thin layer on tortillas, leaving about 1 inch at the bottom. Sprinkle with cheese. Fold bottom of tortilla up about 1 inch, then roll around filling in a cone shape. Fasten with a toothpick and serve. (To serve these piping hot, heat at 425°F for 3 or 4 minutes.)

Yield: 3 servings. These also reheat well in the microwave. One roll-up takes 45 seconds on HIGH.

289 calories per serving, 8.3 g fat (1.2 g saturated), 0 mg cholesterol, 8 g protein, 49 g carbohydrate, 350 mg sodium, 776 mg potassium, 3 mg iron, 5 g fiber, 47 mg calcium. With cheese, 1 serving contains 337 calories, 11.3 g fat (3.1 g saturated) and 169 mg calcium.

■ FISH DISHES

Baked Herbed Fish Fillets

Light, easy and versatile! If you don't have fresh herbs, sprinkle dried herbs over fish. Dried oregano, rosemary and/or thyme are all excellent choices. Balsamic vinegar can be used instead of citrus juice.

> 4 sole, doré or orange roughy fillets (1½ lb/750 g)
> 2 tsp olive or canola oil
> 2 cloves garlic, minced
> 2 tbsp fresh orange, lemon or lime juice
> salt, pepper and paprika, to taste
> 2 tbsp each fresh dill and basil, minced

1. Preheat oven to 425°F. Arrange fish in a single layer on a non-stick or sprayed pan. Brush both sides of fish lightly with oil. Sprinkle evenly with garlic, citrus juice and seasonings. Bake uncovered for 10 to 12 minutes. Fish should flake easily when tested with a fork.

Yield: 4 servings. Do not freeze.

163 calories per serving, 4.1 g fat (0.8 g saturated), 80 mg cholesterol, 29 g protein, 1 g carbohydrate, 124 mg sodium, 433 mg potassium, <1 mg iron, trace fiber, 27 mg calcium.

Variation:
- **Herbed Halibut or Salmon Trout:** *Substitute halibut steaks or salmon trout fillets. Bake 12 to 15 minutes, depending on thickness of fish.*

Easy Pesto Fish Fillets

4 sole or whitefish fillets (1½ lb/750 g)
salt and pepper, to taste
4 tsp Best-O Pesto (see page 149)
2 tbsp grated low-fat mozzarella or Parmesan cheese

1. Preheat oven to 425°F. Line a baking sheet with aluminum foil. Spray
    lightly with non-stick spray. Arrange fish fillets in a single layer and
    sprinkle lightly with salt and pepper. Spread pesto evenly over fish fillets.
    Top with grated cheese. Bake on top rack of oven at 425°F about 10 to
    12 minutes, or until cheese is melted and golden. Fish should flake when
    lightly pressed. (Cooking time may vary slightly, depending on thickness
    of fish.) Serve immediately.

Yield: 4 servings. Do not freeze.

*157 calories per serving, 3.2 g fat (1 g saturated), 82 mg cholesterol, 30 g protein,
trace carbohydrate, 152 mg sodium, 425 mg potassium, <1 mg iron, trace fiber, 55
mg calcium.*

Variation:

*   **Sun-Dried Tomato Pesto Fillets:** *Substitute Sun-Dried Tomato Pesto (see
    page 163).*

Easy Salsa Fish Fillets

This recipe works with any firm-fleshed fish fillets. It's perfect when you're
rushed for time. Serve with basmati rice and lightly steamed green and/or
yellow beans.

4 sole or whitefish fillets (1½ lb/750 g)
salt and pepper, to taste

½ cup bottled salsa (mild or medium)
½ cup grated low-fat mozzarella or cheddar cheese (or ¼ cup grated
Parmesan)

1.   Preheat oven to 425°F. Arrange fish in a single layer on a sprayed foil-
     lined baking pan. Sprinkle with salt and pepper. Top each fillet with 2
     tablespoons of salsa; sprinkle with cheese. Bake uncovered at 425°F for
     10 to 12 minutes, until golden. Fish should flake easily when tested with
     a fork.

Yield: 4 servings. Do not freeze.

*184 calories per serving, 4.3 g fat (2 g saturated), 87 mg cholesterol, 33 g protein,
2 g carbohydrate, 282 mg sodium, 477 mg potassium, <1 mg iron, <1 g fiber, 139
mg calcium.*

Variation:
  • **Salsa Fillets in a Snap:** *Cut several large squares of cooking parchment or
    aluminum foil. Place a fish fillet on each square. Top each one with a spoon-
    ful of Super Salsa (see page 282). Seal packets tightly. Arrange on a baking
    sheet and place in a preheated 400°F oven for 10 to 12 minutes.*

Micropoached Salmon Fillets

A winner in my cooking classes! Other fish fillets (sole, roughy, snapper) can
be used. Salmon is a fatty fish, but very high in omega-3 fatty acids, which
may help fight heart disease. This recipe is so quick and scrumptious, it's no
problem to cook fish two or three times a week!

Romaine or iceberg lettuce leaves
4 salmon fillets, skinned (1.5 lb/750 g)
salt and pepper, to taste

1 tbsp fresh lemon or lime juice
1 tbsp fresh dill, minced (or 1 tsp dried)
additional dill and lemon slices, to garnish

1. Wash lettuce; shake off excess water. Arrange a layer of lettuce leaves in the bottom of a glass pie plate. Arrange fish in a single layer, with thicker edges of fish toward the outside edge of the dish. Season with salt, pepper and lemon juice; top with dill. Cover with another layer of lettuce.
2. Microwave fish on HIGH for 3 minutes. Rotate the plate ¼-turn and cook fish 3 minutes longer. Fish should be even in color. Let fish stand covered for 3 to 4 minutes. It should flake when lightly pressed. If undercooked, microwave 1 or 2 minutes more. Discard lettuce. Garnish salmon with fresh dill and thinly sliced lemon. Delicious hot or cold.

Yield: 4 servings. Leftovers keep 2 or 3 days, or can be frozen to use in casseroles.

246 calories per serving, 11 g fat (1.7 g saturated), 96 mg cholesterol, 34 g protein, trace carbohydrate, 76 mg sodium, 851 mg potassium, 1 mg iron, 0 g fiber, 21 mg calcium.

Notes and Variations:

*   *Even though salmon is considered to be a light choice, portion size is the key! A 3½-ounce portion (100 grams) of salmon contains 177 calories and 7.9 grams of fat. However, most people eat at least double that amount, with double the fat and calories!*
*   *If you don't have a microwave, bake salmon uncovered on a non-stick baking sheet at 450°F for 10 to 12 minutes, or until fish flakes when lightly pressed. (Eliminate lettuce and brush fish lightly with either olive or canola oil or light mayonnaise before cooking to keep it moist.)*
*   *Instead of dill, vary the herbs used to season the fish. Some suggestions are tarragon, parsley, basil, thyme or oregano. If using dried herbs, use one-third the amount.*
*   *Serve salmon with Rainbow Rice Pilaf (see page 204) and steamed broccoli.*

Delicious accompanied with Yogurt Dill Sauce (see page 239) or Dijon Mustard Sauce (see page 122).

- *Salmon Leftovers: Add chunks of poached salmon to Pesto Pasta Salad (see page 108) to turn it into a main dish. Leftover salmon is also delicious mixed with light mayonnaise, minced green onions and celery. Use as a sandwich filling, or serve with mixed greens and garnish with sliced cucumber, tomatoes, minced dill and chives or green onions.*

Pizza Fish Fillets

6 sole fillets (1½ lb/750 g)
salt and pepper, to taste
½ cup pizza or tomato sauce
2 tbsp chopped mushrooms
3 tbsp minced green pepper or zucchini
½ cup grated low-fat mozzarella cheese

1. Preheat oven to 425°F. Spray a foil-lined baking sheet with non-stick spray. Arrange fish in a single layer. Sprinkle lightly with salt and pepper. Spread sauce evenly over fish. Sprinkle with vegetables; top with cheese. Bake uncovered at 425°F for 10 to 12 minutes, or until golden. Fish should flake easily when tested with a fork. Serve immediately.

Yield: 6 servings. Do not freeze.

169 calories per serving, 3.4 g fat (1.5 g saturated), 82 mg cholesterol, 30 g protein, 3 g carbohydrate, 176 mg sodium, 410 mg potassium, <1 mg iron, trace fiber, 90 mg calcium.

Note:

- *Any firm fish can be used (e.g., whitefish, doré or snapper fillets). Halibut steaks can also be used, but increase cooking time to 15 minutes.*

Quick Pickled Salmon

Ready to eat the same day—instead of 4 days later! Pat Brody of Winnipeg shared her recipe with my mom.

2 lb (1 kg) sockeye or cohoe salmon, cut into slices (any fresh salmon can be used)
¾ cup sweet mixed pickles
¾ cup pickle juice
¾ cup ketchup (low-sodium, if available)
1 tbsp mustard seed (or more, to taste)
1 tbsp celery seed (or more, to taste)
2 tbsp sugar
2 tbsp white vinegar
1 onion, chopped
2 carrots, sliced
1 Spanish onion, sliced

1. Rinse fish; drain well. Combine remaining ingredients except Spanish onion and fish in a large pot; bring to a boil. Add fish to hot brine, reduce heat and simmer covered for 7 to 8 minutes. Turn fish over gently and simmer 5 minutes longer.
2. Cool fish slightly, then transfer to a cutting board. Carefully remove skin and center bone. Place Spanish onion slices in an oblong casserole. Put fish on top and cover with brine. When completely cool, cover and refrigerate.

Yield: 6 servings. Delicious hot or cold. Fish keeps a week in the refrigerator or may be frozen.

354 calories per serving, 12.7 g fat (2.2 g saturated), 91 mg cholesterol, 31 g protein, 29 g carbohydrate, 463 mg sodium, 747 mg potassium, 2 mg iron, 3 g fiber, 87 mg calcium.

Note:

- *Pickles, pickle juice and ketchup are high in sodium. Pickle juice is not included in the nutritional analysis; it is used just for marinating the salmon but is not eaten.*

Tuna Caponata

This is similar to ratatouille, but includes tuna, capers and raisins. Vinegar and brown sugar give this versatile vegetarian dish a lovely sweet and sour flavor.

2 lb (1 kg) eggplant, unpeeled
salt, to taste
1 tbsp olive oil
2 medium onions, chopped
2 stalks celery, chopped
1 red pepper, chopped
3 cloves garlic, minced
3 cups mild salsa or tomato sauce
3 tbsp balsamic or red wine vinegar
1 tbsp brown sugar or maple syrup
freshly ground pepper, to taste
1 bay leaf
¼ cup raisins
3 tbsp capers
½ cup pitted sliced black olives
6½ oz can (184 g) water-packed tuna, drained and flaked

1. Cut eggplant into 1-inch pieces. Put into a colander and sprinkle with salt. Place a plate on top of eggplant and top with several cans. Let stand for 30 minutes. Rinse thoroughly. Pat dry with towels.

2.   Spray a large, heavy-bottomed pot with non-stick spray. Add oil and heat on medium-high heat. Sauté onions, celery and red pepper for 5 minutes. Add garlic and eggplant. Sauté a few minutes longer, stirring occasionally. If necessary, add a little water to prevent sticking.

3.   Add remaining ingredients except olives and tuna. Bring to a boil, reduce heat and simmer covered for 25 to 30 minutes, stirring occasionally. Remove from heat and let cool. Stir in olives and tuna. Adjust seasonings to taste. Discard bay leaf. Refrigerate overnight to allow flavors to blend.

Yield: 8 to 10 servings. Keeps about 10 days in the refrigerator, or can be frozen if you omit tuna. Add tuna after Caponata has defrosted.

143 calories per serving, 3.3 g fat (0.5 g saturated), 7 mg cholesterol, 9 g protein, 22 g carbohydrate, 531 mg sodium, 615 mg potassium, 2 mg iron, 6 g fiber, 80 mg calcium.

Notes and Variations:

- *Chef's Serving Suggestions: Place a scoop on a large, fresh leaf of Boston lettuce. Garnish with tomato and cucumber slices. Perfect with any of the previous salads (see pages 93–119)*
- **Stuffed Pasta Shells:** *Use Caponata as a stuffing for cooked jumbo pasta shells. Top with tomato sauce and sprinkle lightly with grated low-fat mozzarella cheese. Bake uncovered at 350°F for 20 minutes, until bubbling hot.*
- *Serve with any of the previous soups above (see pages 82–92).*
- *Caponata makes an excellent vegetable side dish if you omit the tuna. It can also be served as a dip or spread with low GI Pita or low GI crackers, or assorted low GI breads.*

Tuna, Rice and Broccoli Pudding (a.k.a. Kugel)

Excellent for family or friends. It's also perfect for a buffet and wonderful for brunch. Cheese and milk are excellent sources of calcium. Broccoli is a good source of calcium and contains beta carotene.

2 cups water
salt, to taste
1 cup long-grain rice
3 cups broccoli, coarsely chopped
1 onion, chopped
6½ oz can (184 g) tuna, drained and flaked
2 tomatoes, diced
3 eggs plus 2 egg whites
1 cup skim milk
1 cup non-fat or low-fat yogurt
¼ tsp each of basil and oregano
1 cup grated low-fat mozzarella or Swiss cheese
3 tbsp grated Parmesan cheese

1. In a medium saucepan, bring water and a dash of salt to a boil. Add rice, cover and simmer for 20 minutes. (Alternately, microwave rice, water and salt covered on HIGH for 6 to 7 minutes. Reduce power to 50% (MEDIUM); microwave 10 to 12 minutes longer, until water is absorbed.) Let rice stand covered for 10 minutes using either cooking method.

2. Microwave broccoli and onion covered on HIGH for 4 minutes. Let stand covered for 2 minutes. Broccoli should be tender-crisp. Combine with remaining ingredients except Parmesan cheese and mix well. Spread evenly in a lightly greased or sprayed 7 x 11-inch Pyrex casserole. Sprinkle with Parmesan cheese. (Can be prepared in advance up to this point, covered and refrigerated for several hours or overnight.) Bake in a preheated 350°F for 45 minutes, until golden brown.

Yield: 8 servings. Reheats well and/or may be frozen.

212 calories per serving, 3.4 g fat (1.3 g saturated), 89 mg cholesterol, 16 g protein, 29 g carbohydrate, 222 mg sodium, 427 mg potassium, 2 mg iron, 2 g fiber, 171 mg calcium.

Notes and Variations:

- *Use water-packed tuna, not oil-packed. You can use 2 cans of tuna for more protein.*
- *Egg substitute can be used instead of eggs for those with cholesterol problems.*
- ***Salmon, Rice and Broccoli Casserole:*** *Substitute salmon for tuna. (Green beans can replace the broccoli if you like, but then you have to change the name of the recipe!)*

■ CHICKEN AND TURKEY

Curried Chicken, Red Pepper and Mango Salad

This salad is so pretty and it's packed with potassium! Some people are sensitive to mangoes and may develop a red, itchy rash when peeling them. If this applies to you, just wear rubber gloves!

Curried Chicken Salad (see page 141), or 4 cooked skinless chicken breasts, cut in strips
6 cups mixed salad greens
1 mango, peeled
2 red peppers, halved and thinly sliced
1 cup red onion, thinly sliced
½ cup grated carrots
12 cherry tomatoes, halved
2 tbsp balsamic or rice vinegar
1½ tbsp olive oil

½ tbsp sesame oil
2 tbsp orange juice
1 tbsp honey
1 clove garlic, minced
salt and pepper, to taste
2 tbsp toasted slivered almonds, optional

1. Prepare chicken salad (or chicken) as directed. Wash and dry salad greens; arrange on individual plates. Place chicken on greens. Slice mango from the outside through to the middle, saving any juices. Cut away the pit. Arrange sliced mangoes attractively around edge of plate. Garnish with sliced peppers, red onion, carrots and tomatoes. Cover and refrigerate until serving time.
2. Blend vinegar, olive and sesame oils, orange juice, reserved mango juice, honey and garlic. Season with salt and pepper. Drizzle over salad just before serving. Sprinkle with nuts.

Yield: 6 servings.

276 calories per serving, 8 g fat (1.5 g saturated), 64 mg cholesterol, 26 g protein, 26 g carbohydrate, 189 mg sodium, 753 mg potassium, 2 mg iron, 5 g fiber, 75 mg calcium.

Lighter Chicken Salad

Nutritional analysis was done for skinless cooked chicken, using a mixture of light and dark meat. If made with only white meat, one serving will contain 1.3 g fat (0.4 g saturated).

2 cups cooked, diced or chopped chicken
¼ cup minced or grated carrots
2 tbsp minced fresh dill and/or basil (or 1 tsp dried)
2 stalks celery, chopped

4 green onions, chopped
½ of a red pepper, chopped
⅓ cup fat-free or light mayonnaise (approximately)
salt and freshly ground pepper, to taste

1.   Combine all ingredients and mix well. To prepare mixture in your processor, remove and discard skin and bones from chicken. Cut chicken and vegetables into large chunks. First, mince carrots and dill using the Steel Knife. Add celery, green onions and red pepper. Process until chopped. Add chicken and process with quick on/offs, until desired texture is reached. Blend in mayonnaise. Season to taste.

Yield: About 3 cups. Do not freeze.

67 calories per ¼ cup, 2.3 g fat (0.6 g saturated), 27 mg cholesterol, 9 g protein, 2 g carbohydrate, 82 mg sodium, 137 mg potassium, <1 mg iron, <1 g fiber, 14 mg calcium.

Variations:

- ***Curried Chicken Salad:*** *Omit dill and/or basil. One apple, peeled, cored and diced, can be added to the chicken mixture for additional fiber. Season with curry powder to taste.*
- ***Chutney Chicken Salad:*** *Omit dill and/or basil. Add 2 to 3 tablespoons chutney. Add curry powder to taste.*
- ***Oriental Chicken Salad:*** *Omit dill and/or basil. Add ½ cup each drained, chopped water chestnuts, green pepper and/or pineapple tidbits to chicken salad. Blend in 1 to 2 teaspoons soy sauce and a few drops of Oriental sesame oil.*
- ***Honey Mustard Chicken Salad:*** *Blend 2 teaspoons Dijon mustard and 2 teaspoons honey into mayonnaise. Instead of dill or basil, use 1 teaspoon dried thyme or tarragon.*

Lighter Turkey Salad

1.   Substitute cooked turkey breast (or a mixture of white and dark meat) in Lighter Chicken Salad (previous) or any of its variations. (Nutritional analysis is calculated using cooked turkey breast.)

52 calories per ¼ cup, 0.4 g fat (0.1 g saturated), 26 mg cholesterol, 10 g protein, 2 g carbohydrate, 72 mg sodium, 147 mg potassium, <1 mg iron, <1 fiber, 14 mg calcium.

Paul's Carolina Smoked Chicken Salad

My son-in-law Paul Sprackman is an excellent cook! This is one of his extra-special salads. Enjoy!

4 boneless, skinless chicken breasts
2 tsp canola oil
¼ cup dry white wine
1 tsp liquid smoke
8 sun-dried tomatoes (packed in oil), well rinsed, patted dry and cut in strips
2 dozen seedless green grapes, halved
1 medium red onion, chopped
1 green and/or yellow pepper, chopped
¼–⅓ cup low-fat mayonnaise
4–6 drops additional liquid smoke
6–8 drops Tabasco sauce
2–3 tbsp fresh basil, chopped
4 cup mixed salad greens (e.g., mesclun)
¼ cup pecans, coarsely chopped, optional

1.   Marinate chicken in oil, white wine and liquid smoke. Cover and refrigerate overnight. Preheat the grill. Remove chicken from marinade and pat dry. Discard marinade.

2. Grill chicken about 5 to 7 minutes per side. When cool, cut into cubes. In a large bowl, combine chicken with remaining ingredients except salad greens and nuts. Toss gently. Arrange salad greens on individual serving plates. Top with chicken mixture. Sprinkle with pecans, if using.

Yield: 4 to 6 servings.

266 calories per serving, 9.5 g fat (1.7 g saturated), 77 mg cholesterol, 29 g protein, 15 g carbohydrate, 173 mg sodium, 640 mg potassium, 2 mg iron, 2 g fiber, 60 mg calcium.

Rozie's Freeze with Ease Turkey Chili

3 onions, chopped
2 tbsp olive oil, divided
2 cups peppers, chopped (use a mixture of red, green and yellow peppers)
2 cups sliced mushrooms
3–4 cloves garlic, crushed
3 lb minced turkey (preferably turkey breast)
19 oz (540 ml) can red kidney beans
19 oz (540 ml) can white beans
28 oz can (796 ml) puréed Italian tomatoes
3 cups tomato sauce
2-5½ oz cans (156 ml) tomato paste
19 oz (540 ml) can tomato juice
salt and pepper, to taste
2 tbsp chili powder (or to taste)
1 tsp each basil and oregano (or to taste)

1. Spray a large pot with non-stick spray. Heat 1 tablespoon oil on medium heat. Add onions and sauté for 5 to 7 minutes. Add peppers and mushrooms; sauté 5 minutes longer, until tender. Add a little water if

145

veggies begin to stick or burn. Remove veggies from pot and set aside. Heat remaining oil. Add turkey and brown on medium high heat, stirring often. Rinse and drain beans. Add with remaining ingredients to pot. Simmer uncovered for 1 hour, stirring occasionally. Adjust seasonings to taste.

Yield: 15 servings. Reheats and/or freezes well. Freeze in meal-sized batches. Serve over pasta or rice.

285 calories per serving, 3.3 g fat (0.6 g saturated), 66 mg cholesterol, 32 g protein, 34 g carbohydrate, 474 mg sodium, 1164 mg potassium, 4 mg iron, 9 g fiber, 68 mg calcium.

Note:
- *If using cooked turkey, add to chili during last 15 minutes of cooking.*

■ PASTA

PERFECT PASTA-BILITIES
- Pasta has become extremely popular because it is so quick to prepare, requires little fuss or muss, and can be made with just a few simple ingredients from your pantry or freezer.
- The main reason pasta has a bad reputation is due to portion size. Many people eat a heaping plate, thinking sky-high is the limit! Half a cup of cooked pasta is equivalent to 1 starchy choice, the same as a slice of bread. Most people eat 1½ to 2 cups pasta, equal to 3 or 4 slices of bread!
- Another reason many people gain weight from pasta is because of the fat that's added to the sauce! One tablespoon of oil (including olive oil) contains 14 grams of fat. Many recipes contain at least 2 or 3 tablespoons of oil (or more) per serving, while many pasta sauces are loaded with butter and cream (e.g., Alfredo sauce).

- Moderation is the key. Have a bowl of soup and side salad (using a guilt-free dressing) along with your pasta and enjoy your meal without the guilt trip.
- Good news! Research indicates that pasta has a significantly lower glycemic index than bread, thereby having less of an impact on blood sugar. People who are carb sensitive can enjoy pasta in moderation, but should probably minimize their consumption of all high GI breads.
- Experiment with different pastas and sauces to experience a quick trip around the world without leaving the comfort of your home.
- It's fun to use different shapes. Try shells, wagon wheels, bow ties, orzo, traditional or whole grain spaghetti, fettucine or angel hair pasta. Bulk stores have a wonderful selection, from spicy penne to spinach linguine, plus many pastas made from a variety of grains (e.g., Chinese cellophane noodles made from mung beans, soba noodles made from buckwheat, rice noodles, quinoa spirals, vegetable shells). Experiment and enjoy.
- Read labels before you buy. Choose enriched high-quality pasta made exclusively with hard (durum) wheat as it has more protein and less starch. Another excellent choice is whole-wheat pasta made from durum whole-wheat semolina, as it's low in fat and high in fiber. If you can't find the shape called for in a recipe, use a similar type.
- To cook pasta, use a large pot and 4 to 5 quarts (liters) of water for each pound (500 grams) of pasta. Don't add oil to the cooking water, but add a little salt if you are not on a salt-restricted diet. The glycemic index of pasta is lower when cooked al dente, because it's digested more slowly, preventing spikes in blood sugar.
- Noodles swell slightly when cooked; spaghetti and macaroni double in volume. Allow about 2 ounces of dried pasta as a side dish, 3 to 4 ounces as a main dish. It depends on what other ingredients are combined with the pasta, as well as the rest of your menu.

- I used to rinse cooked pasta, but don't any more, except for recipes like noodle kugel. Rinsing removes the starch that helps the sauce cling to the pasta.
- Save a little of the cooking water and mix it together with the pasta and sauce. It will act as a thickener, preventing the pasta from sitting in a puddle of water on the serving plate!
- In a hurry? A simple tomato sauce is always a great choice, either store-bought or homemade. For variety, add a handful of leftovers, such as cooked chicken, fish or vegetables. Other ideas are tofu, canned beans or chickpeas, herbs, garlic, onions, sun-dried tomatoes, frozen vegetables (e.g., broccoli, cauliflower, snow peas), sautéed mushrooms and/or onions.
- Add a little olive oil to tomato sauce for a healthy helping of lycopene, which has anti-cancer properties. Lycopene is more readily available from cooked tomatoes, not raw, and needs fat to be absorbed. Top with a sprinkling of freshly grated Parmesan cheese for a simple, delicious meal.
- Cooked pasta reheats beautifully in the microwave. Allow 1 minute on HIGH per cup of pasta.
- Most pasta dishes freeze well, so why not double the recipe? Pack leftovers in individual containers, seal tightly, label and freeze. You'll have frozen dinners that taste better (and are better for you!) than expensive packaged meals in the supermarket freezer.
- Timesaving Secret: Cook extra pasta, rinse, drain and cool. Freeze portions in ziploc bags. When needed, remove pasta from bag, place in a strainer and rinse with hot water. Ready to serve with your favorite sauce! Thanks to my well-organized assistant Elaine Kaplan for the super tip!
- If you eat out frequently, make friends with the restaurant manager. Phone ahead and explain your needs. Most restaurants are glad to help. They need customers who will be around (not round!) for a long time.
- So, wise up and you'll lighten up! Cut the fat, add some veggies and don't pass up the pasta.

Best-O Pesto

My original recipe had 83 calories and over 8 grams of fat per tablespoon. This lighter version has a fraction of the fat!

2 tbsp pine nuts (or walnuts)
2 cups tightly packed fresh basil leaves
½ cup fresh parsley
4 cloves garlic, peeled
2–3 tbsp grated Parmesan cheese
2 tbsp olive oil (extra-virgin is best)
¼ cup tomato juice or vegetable broth
salt and pepper, to taste

1. Place nuts in a small skillet and brown over medium heat for 2 to 3 minutes. Wash basil and parsley; dry thoroughly. Start the food processor and drop garlic through feed tube. Process until minced. Add nuts, basil, parsley and Parmesan cheese. Process until fine, about 15 seconds. Drizzle oil and juice through the feed tube while the machine is running. Process until blended. Season to taste.

Yield: 1 cup. Pesto keeps for 4–5 days in the refrigerator, or can be frozen for 2 months.

27 calories per tbsp, 2.4 g fat (0.5 g saturated), <1 mg cholesterol, <1 g protein, <1 g carbohydrate, 30 mg sodium, 52 mg potassium, trace iron, trace fiber, 23 mg calcium.

Notes:
- *When basil is expensive, use a combination of fresh basil and fresh spinach. It works perfectly!*
- *Freeze pesto in ice cube trays. Transfer them to a plastic bag and store in the freezer. Each cube contains 2 tablespoons pesto. Add a cube or two to your favorite pasta sauce, soup or vegetarian stew.*
- *A couple of spoonfuls of pesto added to pasta salad or vinaigrette dressing will enhance the flavor.*

Cheater's Hi-Fiber Pasta Sauce

Great when you're in a hurry. Just combine a can of lentils, a jar of sauce and a splash of wine. Yum!

> 1 cup cooked lentils (or canned, rinsed and well-drained)
> 1 jar vegetarian spaghetti sauce (about 3 cups)
> ¼ cup water
> 1–2 tbsp red or white wine, if desired

1. Process lentils in your food processor until puréed. Add spaghetti sauce and process until well mixed, scraping down sides of bowl as needed. Combine puréed mixture with water and wine (if using) in a large sauce pan. Bring to a boil and simmer partially covered for 10 minutes (or microwave uncovered on HIGH for 10 minutes), stirring occasionally.

Yield: About 4 cups sauce. Freezes and/or reheats well.

101 calories per ½ cup serving, 3.7 g fat (0.5 g saturated), 0 mg cholesterol, 4 g protein, 15 g carbohydrate, 499 mg sodium, 521 mg potassium, 2 mg iron, 4 g fiber, 29 mg calcium.

Notes and Variations:

- *If using this sauce in dishes which require further cooking, don't bother precooking the sauce.*
- *To use sauce over spaghetti, simmer the sauce while pasta is cooking. If desired, stir some frozen mixed vegetables into the sauce for extra nutrients. They'll defrost and cook with the sauce!*
- *If you have time, sauté some onions, peppers, mushrooms and/or zucchini in a little olive oil or vegetable broth. Combine veggies with sauce ingredients and simmer uncovered for 10 minutes.*

Cheater's Pasta

This quick and easy recipe comes from Sharon Druker, a former student with a very busy lifestyle!

1 lb (454 g) spaghetti or linguini
28 oz can (796 ml) Italian chopped seasoned tomatoes
1 tsp chopped garlic in oil
½ tsp dried basil (to taste)
½ tsp dried oregano (to taste)
6½ oz can (184 g) water-packed tuna, drained and flaked
1 to 2 tsp capers
¼ to ½ cup sliced black olives, optional

1. Cook pasta according to package directions. Drain but do not rinse. While pasta is cooking, put canned tomatoes, garlic and oil in a large pot. Add seasonings and heat to simmering. Add tuna and capers. Simmer just until heated through. Place pasta on serving plates and top with sauce. Garnish with olives if desired.

Yield: 6 servings. Do not freeze.

410 calories per serving, 0.7 g fat (0.1 g saturated), 9 mg cholesterol, 27 g protein, 71 g carbohydrate, 437 mg sodium, 159 mg potassium, 3 mg iron, 5 g fiber, 74 mg calcium.

Fasta Pasta

This is a great last-minute dish to make when you're rushed for time.

2 cups rotini or macaroni
1 onion, chopped
2 tsp canola oil
1 lb extra-lean ground turkey, chicken or beef
2½ cups bottled marinara/spaghetti sauce

½ cup water
3 cups frozen mixed vegetables
salt, pepper and garlic powder, to taste

1. Cook pasta in boiling, salted water according to package directions.
Drain and rinse; set aside. Meanwhile, spray a large pot with non-stick
spray. Sauté onion briefly in oil. Add meat and brown for 6 to 8 minutes,
stirring often. Remove excess fat from browned meat mixture by placing
it in a fine strainer and rinsing it quickly under running water. Return
meat to pan along with tomato sauce, water and frozen vegetables. Cover
and simmer for 15 minutes, stirring occasionally. Stir in pasta and cook 5
minutes longer, until heated through. Season to taste.

Yield: 6 servings. Leftovers will keep for a day or 2 in the refrigerator or can
be frozen.

*357 calories per serving, 7 g fat (0.9 g saturated), 55 mg cholesterol, 28 g protein,
48 g carbohydrate, 615 mg sodium, 877 mg potassium, 4 mg iron, 8 g fiber, 68
mg calcium.*

Hi-Fiber Vegetarian Lasagna

For smaller families, make several smaller lasagnas in loaf pans and freeze
them. So handy!

4 cups Hi-Fiber Vegetarian Pasta Sauce (see page 152) or Cheater's
High-Fiber Pasta Sauce (see page 150)
9 lasagna noodles, cooked, drained and laid flat on towels
2 cups low-fat Ricotta or dry cottage cheese
1½ to 2 cups grated low-fat Mozzarella cheese
6 tbsp grated Parmesan cheese

1. Place about ⅓ of the sauce in the bottom of a lightly greased or sprayed 9 x 13-inch casserole. Arrange 3 lasagna noodles in a single layer over sauce. Top with ½ of the Ricotta, ⅓ of the mozzarella and ½ of the Parmesan. Repeat with sauce, noodles and cheese. Top with noodles, sauce and mozzarella cheese. (Can be made in advance up to this point and refrigerated or frozen. Thaw before cooking.) Bake uncovered in a preheated 375°F oven for 40 to 45 minutes. Let stand for 10 to 15 minutes for easier cutting.

Yield: 10 to 12 servings. Freezes and/or reheats well.

271 calories per serving, 9.3 g fat (5.2 g saturated), 27 mg cholesterol, 18 g protein, 30 g carbohydrate, 239 mg sodium, 408 mg potassium, 2 mg iron, 5 g fiber, 328 mg calcium.

Notes:
- *Fresh lasagna noodles or no-cook packaged noodles can be used. No need to precook them!*
- *Dry cottage cheese is more difficult to spread than ricotta, so thin it with a few drops of skim milk. If using creamed cottage cheese, purée it in the processor for 2 to 3 minutes, until smooth.*
- *Don't fuss too much about spreading the cheese evenly. Drop it by spoonfuls over the noodles. Don't worry if there are any spaces. The cheese will spread during baking.*

Kasha and Bow Ties with Mushrooms

Use gourmet mushrooms to bring this old-fashioned recipe to new heights. Kasha (buckwheat groats) is one of my favorite foods. It's rich in protein, particularly lysine, as well as iron, calcium and B vitamins. I love knowing that kasha is so good for me!

2 cups bow-tie pasta (3-color or mini bow ties)
1 cup medium or coarse kasha
1 egg white
2 cups hot chicken or vegetable broth
salt and pepper, to taste
1 tbsp canola or olive oil
2 large onions, coarsely chopped
2 cups sliced mushrooms (Portobello, shiitake, oyster or button mushrooms)
½ cup chopped red pepper, if desired
2–3 tbsp minced fresh dill

1. Cook pasta in boiling, salted water according to package directions. Drain and rinse well. In a large heavy-bottomed pot, mix kasha with egg white. Cook on medium heat, stirring constantly, until kasha is dry and toasted, about 5 minutes. Remove pan from heat and slowly add broth to kasha. Return pan to heat, cover and simmer for 10 to 12 minutes, until most of liquid is absorbed. Holes will appear on the surface and kasha should be tender. Remove from heat and let stand covered for a few minutes, until remaining liquid is absorbed. Fluff with a fork. Season with salt and pepper.

2. Heat oil in a large non-stick skillet. Add onions and sauté on medium-high heat for 7 to 8 minutes, until nicely browned. If necessary, add a little water or broth as needed to prevent sticking. Add mushrooms and red pepper. Cook a few minutes longer, until golden, stirring occasionally. Combine all ingredients and mix well. Adjust seasonings to taste.

Yield: 8 servings. Freezes and/or reheats well. Recipe can be doubled easily.

148 calories per serving, 2.4 g fat (0.2 g saturated), 0 mg cholesterol, 6 g protein, 26 g carbohydrate, 59 mg sodium, 150 mg potassium, 2 mg iron, 2 g fiber, 19 mg calcium.

Variations:

- *For vegetarians who don't eat eggs, use no-egg pasta. For those with celiac disease, pastas based on stone-ground buckwheat or soy flour are acceptable in terms of both GI and celiac disease. Gluten is a protein found in wheat, rye and barley products.*
- *For a light and fluffy texture, use ¾ cup kasha and ¼ cup bulgur. Instead of mixing kasha with an egg white, brown it in 1 tablespoon additional oil. If cooked kasha seems dry, moisten it with additional broth before serving.*
- ***Kasha Pilaf with Squash:*** *Prepare kasha as directed above, but omit pasta. Pierce an acorn squash all over with the point of a sharp knife. Microwave on HIGH for 6 to 8 minutes, turning it over halfway through cooking. Let stand for 10 minutes. Test with a knife; it should pass through the squash easily. Cut squash in half, discard seeds and cut into ½-inch cubes. Add to kasha along with sautéed onions, mushrooms and dill. Add salt and pepper to taste*

Mexican Pasta with Beans
Full of fiber, full of beans, full of flavor!

2 tsp olive oil
1 onion, chopped
2 cloves garlic, crushed
1 green or red pepper, chopped
1 jalapeño or chili pepper, seeded and minced
19 oz (540 ml) can kidney or black beans, rinsed and drained
28 oz (796 ml) can diced tomatoes
salt and pepper, to taste
½ tsp oregano
1 lb spaghetti, penne or rotini
¼ cup chopped coriander (cilantro)
¼ cup chopped green onions, to garnish
grated low-fat cheddar cheese, optional

1. Heat oil in a non-stick skillet. Sauté onion, garlic and peppers for 5 minutes. Add beans, tomatoes, salt, pepper and oregano. Simmer uncovered for 10 to 15 minutes, stirring occasionally. Meanwhile, cook pasta according to package directions. Drain well but do not rinse, reserving ½ to ¾ cup of the cooking water. Mix pasta with sauce and reserved cooking water. Serve on hot plates. Garnish with coriander and green onions. If desired, sprinkle lightly with grated cheese.

Yield: 6 servings. Sauce can be frozen.

456 calories per serving, 2.4 g fat (0.3 g saturated), 0 mg cholesterol, 24 g protein, 83 g carbohydrate, 12 mg sodium, 149 mg potassium, 2 mg iron, 12 g fiber, 31 mg calcium.

Note:
- *Wear rubber gloves or put plastic bags on your hands when handling hot peppers. The smaller the pepper, the hotter it is. Don't rub your eyes or touch sensitive body parts after handling peppers.*

Penne Al Pesto Jardinière

The starchy cooking liquid binds with the cheese to thicken the sauce. So pretty with 3-color pasta!

1 lb penne (ziti, fusilli or rotini can be used)
1 onion, halved and cut in strips
4 peppers, (green, red, yellow and/or orange), halved, seeded and cut in strips
2 zucchini, cut in strips
3 cloves garlic, crushed
1½ tbsp olive oil
3–4 tbsp balsamic vinegar or lemon juice
salt and pepper, to taste

¼ cup grated Parmesan cheese
½ cup fresh basil, finely chopped
1½–2 cups tomato sauce (bottled or homemade)
1 chopped tomato, to garnish
Parmesan cheese, to garnish

1. Preheat oven to 425°F. Prepare vegetables and place on a sprayed (or non-stick) baking sheet. Add garlic, olive oil and vinegar. Sprinkle lightly with salt and pepper and mix well. Roast vegetables uncovered at 425°F for 20 minutes, until nicely browned.
2. Meanwhile, bring a large pot of salted water to a boil. Cook pasta according to package directions, about 10 minutes, until al dente. Ladle out a little of the cooking liquid just before draining pasta. Drain pasta but do not rinse.
3. Return pasta to saucepan. Add Parmesan, basil and about ¼ cup of reserved cooking liquid; mix well. Add tomato sauce and roasted vegetables. Adjust seasonings to taste. Cook briefly, just until heated through. Garnish with diced tomato and sprinkle with a light dusting of Parmesan cheese, if desired. Great hot or at room temperature.

Yield: 8 main dish servings. Reheats well. If frozen, vegetables may lose some of their texture.

267 calories per serving, 4.6 g fat (1.1 g saturated), 3 mg cholesterol, 9 g protein, 48 g carbohydrate, 342 mg sodium, 434 mg potassium, 3 mg iron, 4 g fiber, 77 mg calcium.

Variation:

- **Penne with Roasted Vegetable Purée:** *In Step 2, reserve about a cup of the cooking liquid from pasta. In Step 3, process 2 cups of the roasted vegetables until smooth. Add ½ cup of reserved cooking liquid to thin the mixture; process briefly. (If necessary, add a little more liquid.) Stir purée into pasta along with remaining ingredients. (This is a great way to get kids to eat their veggies!)*

157

Penne with Roasted Peppers and Sun-Dried Tomatoes

The tomato sauce is used to moisten the pasta and give it a hint of color.

1 pkg (1 lb/500 g) penne or other pasta
1 cup jarred roasted red peppers, cut in strips
½ cup sun-dried tomatoes
2 medium onions, chopped (or cut in strips)
1 tbsp olive oil
1 zucchini, sliced (optional)
3 cloves garlic, minced
⅓ cup fresh basil, finely chopped
¼ cup grated Parmesan cheese
1½–2 cups tomato sauce
salt and pepper, to taste

1. Set a large pot of water up to boil for the pasta. Meanwhile, roast peppers as directed. Cut them into strips. Soak sun-dried tomatoes in boiling water for 10 to 15 minutes, until rehydrated. Drain and dry well; cut into strips.

2. Sauté onions in olive oil on medium heat for 3 to 4 minutes. Add zucchini and garlic; cook 3 to 4 minutes longer. If necessary, add a little water to prevent burning. Cook pasta in boiling salted water for 10 to 12 minutes, until al dente. Drain well. Combine all ingredients and mix well. Delicious hot or at room temperature.

Yield: 6 servings. Reheats and freezes well. If necessary, add a little extra tomato sauce when reheating.

343 calories per serving, 5.2 g fat (1.4 g saturated), 3 mg cholesterol, 13 g protein, 62 g carbohydrate, 683 mg sodium, 509 mg potassium, 4 mg iron, 5 g fiber, 100 mg calcium.

Notes and Variations:

- *If using roasted peppers from the jar, drain and rinse them thoroughly to remove excess sodium.*
- *Chef's Shortcut! Instead of soaking the sun-dried tomatoes, add them along with the pasta to the boiling water. They will rehydrate by the time the pasta has cooked!*
- ***Pasta with Mushrooms, Roasted Peppers and Sun-Dried Tomatoes:*** *Soak ¼ to ⅓ cup of dried exotic mushrooms (e.g. porcini, shiitake) in boiling water to cover. (Soak them separately from the sun-dried tomatoes. The soaking liquid from mushrooms can be added to your favorite vegetable broth to enhance the flavor.) Add drained mushrooms to the onions along with zucchini and garlic; sauté for 3 or 4 minutes.*

Quick 'n Easy Tomato Sauce (Vegetarian Spaghetti Sauce)

This sauce is a quick and easy substitute for the bottled version! To make it fat-free, omit olive oil.

28 oz can (796 ml) tomatoes (stewed, whole or crushed)
5½ oz can (156 ml) tomato paste
1 tsp olive oil (preferably extra-virgin)
3 cloves garlic, crushed
salt and pepper, to taste
¼ tsp cayenne or red pepper flakes
½ tsp oregano
1 tbsp fresh basil, minced (or ½ tsp dried)
½ tsp sugar
1–2 tbsp red or white wine, optional

1. Combine all ingredients in a large saucepan or covered microsafe casserole, breaking up tomatoes if necessary. To microwave, cook covered on HIGH for 10 minutes, stirring at half time. To cook conventionally,

bring sauce to a boil, reduce heat and simmer covered for 20 to 25 minutes, stirring occasionally. Adjust seasonings to taste.

Yield: Approximately 4 cups sauce. Reheats and/or freezes well. Freeze in 1 cup portions.

43 calories per ½ cup serving, 0.8 g fat (0.1 g saturated), 0 mg cholesterol, 2 g protein, 9 g carbohydrate, 27 mg sodium, 413 mg potassium, 1 mg iron, 2 g fiber, 40 mg calcium.

Notes and Variations:

- *If you're sodium-sensitive, use canned tomatoes and tomato paste without added salt.*
- ***Sun-Dried Tomato Sauce:*** *Soak ½ cup sun-dried tomatoes (dry pack) in boiling water for 10 minutes, until soft. Drain well; chop coarsely. Add to sauce ingredients and cook as directed.*
- ***Light 'n Easy Meat Sauce:*** *Sauté 1 onion, 1 green pepper and 2 cloves crushed garlic in 2 tablespoons water until tender (or microwave on HIGH for 3 minutes). Add 1 pound lean ground turkey and cook until it loses its pink color, stirring occasionally (about 5 to 6 minutes in the microwave). Add remaining ingredients and simmer covered for about 1 hour (or 20 minutes on HIGH in the microwave). Stir occasionally. Adjust seasonings to taste. Makes about 6 cups of sauce. Half a cup of sauce contains about 91 calories and 3.7 grams fat (1 gram saturated).*
- *Fiber Facts: Add a finely grated carrot to the sauce for fiber and natural sweetness.*
- *Most pasta sauces freeze beautifully. Pack in 1 cup containers for convenience, leaving about half an inch space at the top to allow for expansion. When you need some sauce, place the frozen container under running water briefly. Pop out the contents and transfer them to a microsafe bowl. Thaw on HIGH power. (DEFROST takes too long!) Stir several times. One cup of sauce takes about 5 minutes to thaw and heat.*

Roasted Tomato, Garlic and Basil Sauce

Roasting brings out the flavor of the vegetables. This sauce is simply the best!

2 dozen Italian plum tomatoes (3 lb/1.4 kg)
2 onions, peeled
1 large red pepper, seeded
6–8 cloves garlic, peeled
1–2 tbsp extra-virgin olive oil
¼–½ cup fresh basil, to taste
salt and pepper, to taste

1. Preheat oven to 400°F. Core tomatoes and cut in half lengthwise. Cut onions and red pepper into chunks. Arrange in a single layer on a non-stick baking sheet along with garlic. Drizzle lightly with oil. Roast uncovered at 400°F for 45 to 50 minutes, or until vegetables are soft and lightly browned.
2. Combine roasted vegetables with basil in the processor. (You may have to do this in 2 batches.) Process until fairly smooth. Season to taste with salt and pepper.

Yield: About 4 cups sauce (8 servings of about ½ cup). Reheats and/or freezes well. (It's a great idea to make a double or triple batch!)

78 calories per ½ cup serving, 2.5 g fat (0.4 g saturated), 0 mg cholesterol, 2 g protein, 14 g carbohydrate, 21 mg sodium, 548 mg potassium, 1 mg iron, 3 g fiber, 23 mg calcium.

Note:
  • *You can roast other vegetables along with the tomatoes. Try zucchini, eggplant, mushrooms and/or green pepper. Cut vegetables in chunks before cooking. Process the cooked vegetables with basil using quick on/offs, until desired texture is reached.*

Simple 'n Spicy Spirals
Simply wonderful when you're in a hurry!

> 3 cup bottled salsa (mild or medium)
> 1 lb (500 g) spirals (or bow-tie pasta)
> 1 cup grated low-fat mozzarella cheese

1. Prepare salsa as directed and heat it until piping hot. Meanwhile, cook pasta according to package directions. Drain pasta but do not rinse. Return pasta to the pot. Mix pasta with some of the hot salsa to lightly coat pasta; mix well. Place on serving plates. Top with additional salsa; sprinkle lightly with cheese. It will melt from the heat of the pasta and salsa. (Or heat it in the microwave on HIGH for about a minute.) Serve immediately. Perfect with a large garden salad.

Yield: 6 servings. Reheats and/or freezes well.

351 calories per serving, 4.5 g fat (2.2 g saturated), 10 mg cholesterol, 16 g protein, 60 g carbohydrate, 566 mg sodium, 158 mg potassium, 4 mg iron, 4 g fiber, 190 mg calcium.

Variation:
- ***Greek-Style Pasta:*** *Use crumbled feta cheese instead of mozzarella. Prepare Simple Salsa but don't heat it. Combine cooked, drained pasta, salsa and feta cheese. Serve at room temperature.*

Spaghetti with Roasted Tomato, Garlic and Basil Sauce

> Roasted Tomato, Garlic and Basil Sauce (see page 161)
> 1 lb (500 g) enriched spaghetti
> Grated Parmesan cheese, optional

1. Prepare sauce and keep it warm. Cook pasta according to package directions. Drain, reserving about ½ cup of the cooking water in the pot. Do not rinse pasta. Return pasta to the pot. Add just enough of the sauce to lightly coat the pasta; mix well. Place on serving plates. Serve with additional sauce. Sprinkle with a little grated Parmesan cheese, if desired.

Yield: 6 servings. Reheats and/or freezes well, providing sauce was not previously frozen.

321 calories per serving, 2.8 g fat (0.4 g saturated), 0 mg cholesterol, 16 g protein, 60 g carbohydrate, 28 mg sodium, 610 mg potassium, 2 mg iron, 6 g fiber, 38 mg calcium.

Sun-Dried Tomato Pesto

½ cup sun-dried tomatoes (dry-pack)
⅓ cup tightly packed fresh basil leaves
½ cup parsley
4–5 large cloves garlic
2 tbsp finely ground almonds
3 tbsp grated Parmesan cheese
2 tbsp olive oil (preferably extra-virgin)
½ cup tomato juice

1. Cover sun-dried tomatoes with boiling water. Let stand for 20 minutes, until rehydrated. Drain well. Rinse basil and parsley; dry well. Start the processor and drop garlic through feed tube. Process until minced. Add sun-dried tomatoes, basil, parsley, almonds and Parmesan cheese. Process until fine, about 15 to 20 seconds. Add olive oil and tomato juice and process until well blended, scraping down sides of bowl as necessary.

Yield: About 1½ cups. Pesto will keep for 4 or 5 days in the refrigerator, or can be frozen for up to 2 months.

31 calories per tbsp, 2.2 g fat (0.4 g saturated), <1 mg cholesterol, 1 g protein, 2 g carbohydrate, 99 mg sodium, 130 mg potassium, <1 mg iron, <1 g fiber, 23 mg calcium.

Vegetarian Pad Thai

So yummy! It was very difficult to slash the fat from the original recipe. This version is much lower in fat, but if you don't watch your portion size, you'll be calling this dish "padded thighs!"

fish sauce* (see directions following the recipe)
2 tsp Worcestershire sauce
3 tbsp sugar
¼ cup fresh lime juice (from 3 or 4 limes)
10 oz pkg extra-firm silken tofu, cut in 1" cubes (1% fat)
12 oz flat rice noodles (or fettucine)
1 tbsp canola oil
2–3 cloves garlic, crushed
6 green onions, sliced
1 cup red pepper strips
¼ tsp red pepper flakes
3–4 tbsp chopped peanuts, divided
2 cup bean sprouts
¼ cup fresh coriander/cilantro, minced (to garnish)
1 red chili pepper, seeded and minced (to garnish)

1. Prepare fish sauce as directed. Combine with Worcestershire sauce, sugar and lime juice in a bowl. Add tofu cubes and marinate for 1 hour at room temperature or up to 8 hours in the refrigerator. Drain, reserving marinade.
2. If using rice noodles, soak in 6 cups of hot water until soft, about 1 hour. Discard water. If using fettucine, cook according to package directions. Drain well. Set aside.

3.　　Assembly: Use a large non-stick wok or skillet. Spray lightly with non-stick spray. Heat oil. Add garlic, green onions and red pepper strips. Sauté for 2 to 3 minutes on medium-high heat. Add red pepper flakes, drained tofu and 1 tablespoon of peanuts. Stir-fry 2 to 3 minutes longer. Add bean sprouts, reserved marinade and drained noodles. Stir-fry until heated through. Garnish with remaining peanuts, coriander and chilis. Serve immediately.

Yield: 4 to 6 servings. Do not freeze.

499 calories per serving, 9 g fat (1.5 g saturated), 5 mg cholesterol, 19 g protein, 87 g carbohydrate, 536 mg sodium, 461 mg potassium, 4 mg iron, 2 g fiber, 92 mg calcium.

** **Fish Sauce**: Commercial fish sauce is usually made from shrimp, salt and water. It can be found in Oriental groceries. An acceptable substitute can be made from 6 anchovy fillets, well rinsed and drained. Mash together with 1 clove of crushed garlic and 1 tablespoon soy sauce. It works beautifully in this recipe.*

■ VEGETABLE DISHES

Belle's Chunky Ratatouille
This is my mother's recipe for ratatouille. It's addictive!

　　2 onions, thinly sliced
　　1 tbsp olive oil
　　3 cloves garlic, crushed
　　1 small eggplant (about ¾ lb/340 g), cut in chunks
　　1 green pepper, cut in strips
　　2 red peppers, cut in strips
　　1 jalapeño pepper, finely chopped (optional)
　　2 medium zucchini, sliced

2 large ripe tomatoes, cut into chunks

8 oz can (237 ml) tomato sauce

1 tbsp balsamic vinegar

salt and pepper, to taste

pinch of chili flakes

⅛ tsp chili powder

⅛ tsp oregano

⅛ tsp mixed Italian seasoning

⅛ tsp cumin, optional

1 tsp sugar

2 tbsp fresh basil, chopped (or 1 tsp dried)

1. Sauté onions in oil on medium heat for 3 or 4 minutes. Add garlic and sauté briefly. Add eggplant. Sauté for 5 minutes longer, stirring occasionally. Add peppers and zucchini; sauté for 5 minutes. Add remaining ingredients. Bring to a boil, reduce heat and simmer covered for 25 minutes longer, until vegetables are tender. Stir occasionally. Tastes even better when reheated.

Yield: 6 to 8 servings. This keeps 7 to 10 days in the refrigerator. Freezes well.

112 calories per serving, 3.1 g fat (0.5 g saturated), 0 mg cholesterol, 4 g protein, 21 g carbohydrate, 241 mg sodium, 801 mg potassium, 2 mg iron, 5 g fiber, 49 mg calcium.

Black Bean and Corn Casserole

Elegant enough for guests. Serve over rice or pasta with Israeli Salad (see page 103), or use as a side dish. Full of fiber, full of beans!

4 cups cooked or canned black beans

2 cups stewed tomatoes or tomato sauce

3 tbsp maple syrup or brown sugar

2 medium onions, chopped
1 green pepper, chopped
1 red pepper, chopped
¾ cup canned or frozen corn niblets
1 tsp Dijon mustard
½ tsp each cayenne pepper and chili powder
freshly ground pepper, to taste

1. Spray a 2-quart ovenproof casserole with non-stick spray. Combine all ingredients and mix well. Bake covered at 350°F for 45 minutes, until bubbling hot and flavors are blended. (Or microwave in a covered microsafe casserole on HIGH for 15 to 18 minutes. Stir once or twice during cooking.)

Yield: 6 servings of about 1 cup each. Freezes and/or reheats well. Also delicious cold.

207 calories per cup, 1 g fat (0.2 g saturated), 0 mg cholesterol, 10 g protein, 42 g carbohydrate, 270 mg sodium, 577 mg potassium, 3 mg iron, 10 g fiber, 62 mg calcium.

Broccoli Noodle Pudding (a.k.a. Kugel)

Mimi Brownstein gave me the idea for this luscious kugel. It's perfect for a buffet or dinner party!

12 oz pkg (375 g) medium noodles
1 bunch broccoli (about 1 lb/500 g)
2 tsp canola oil
2 onions, chopped
1 red pepper, chopped
2 cloves garlic, crushed
1 cup mushrooms, sliced

167

3 eggs plus 4 egg whites (5 eggs or 1¼ cups egg substitute can be used)
2 cups chicken or vegetable broth
salt and pepper, to taste

1. Preheat oven to 350°F. Cook noodles according to package directions. Drain and rinse well. Soak broccoli in cold water for 10 minutes. Drain well. Cut broccoli into florets; slice the stems. Steam or microwave the broccoli covered on HIGH for 5 minutes, until tender-crisp.
2. Heat oil in a non-stick skillet. Sauté onions, red pepper and garlic on medium-high heat until golden, about 5 minutes. (If needed, add a little water or broth to prevent sticking.) Add mushrooms and sauté 4 or 5 minutes longer. Combine all ingredients and mix well. Spread evenly in a sprayed 9 x 13-inch casserole. Bake at 350°F for 30 minutes. Cover with foil and bake 30 minutes longer. Cool for 10 minutes before slicing into squares.

Yield: 12 servings. Freezes and/or reheats well.

173 calories per serving, 3.6 g fat (0.9 g saturated), 87 mg cholesterol, 10 g protein, 26 g carbohydrate, 102 mg sodium, 262 mg potassium, 2 mg iron, 3 g fiber, 52 mg calcium.

Easy Enchiladas

1 onion, chopped
1 cup mushrooms, sliced
2 tsp olive oil
2 cloves garlic, crushed
19 oz (540 ml) can kidney beans
1 cup canned or frozen corn, drained
2 cups tomato sauce

¼ tsp red pepper flakes
8 flour tortillas
1 cup grated low-fat cheddar cheese

1. Preheat oven to 350°F. Sauté onion and mushrooms in oil for 5 minutes. Add garlic and cook 2 minutes longer. Rinse and drain beans thoroughly. Place beans in a bowl and mash slightly. Add to skillet along with corn. Add ½ cup of sauce and red pepper flakes; mix well.
2. Spray an oblong Pyrex casserole with non-stick spray. Soften tortillas by heating in the microwave on HIGH about 1 minute. Spread ½ cup sauce in bottom of casserole. Spoon some of bean/corn mixture on each tortilla in a strip across the middle. Roll up tightly and arrange seam side down in casserole. Top with remaining sauce. Cover and bake for 25 minutes. Uncover, sprinkle with cheese and bake uncovered 5 to 10 minutes longer, until cheese is melted.

Yield: 8 enchiladas. These reheat and/or freeze well.

199 calories per serving, 5 g fat (1.1 g saturated), 3 mg cholesterol, 11 g protein, 30 g carbohydrate, 508 mg sodium, 346 mg potassium, 1 mg iron, 5 g fiber, 105 mg calcium.

Easy Vegetarian Chili
You won't believe this delicious, high-fiber chili contains no meat! Don't be deterred by the long list of ingredients. They're mostly herbs and spices. This chili is quick to prepare and tastes better the next day! Cocoa is the secret ingredient. It deepens the color and rounds out the flavor.

1 tbsp olive or canola oil
2 onions, chopped
2 green and/or red peppers, chopped
3 cloves garlic, crushed

2 cups mushrooms, sliced
2 cups cooked or canned red kidney beans
2 cups cooked or canned chickpeas
½ cup bulgur or couscous, rinsed
28 oz (796 ml) can tomatoes (or 6 fresh tomatoes, chopped)
1 cup bottled salsa (mild or medium)
½ cup water
1 tsp salt (or to taste)
1 tbsp chili powder
1 tsp dried basil
½ tsp each pepper, oregano and cumin
¼ tsp cayenne
1 tbsp unsweetened cocoa powder
1 tsp sugar
1 cup corn niblets, optional

- *Conventional Method:* Heat oil in a large pot. Sauté onions, peppers and garlic for 5 minutes on medium heat. Add mushrooms and sauté 4 or 5 minutes more. Add remaining ingredients except corn. Bring to a boil and simmer, covered, for 25 minutes, stirring occasionally. Stir in corn.
- *Microwave Method:* Combine oil, onions, peppers and garlic in a 3-quart microsafe pot. Microwave covered on HIGH for 5 minutes. Add mushrooms and microwave 2 minutes longer. Add remaining ingredients except corn. Cover and microwave on HIGH for 18 to 20 minutes, stirring once or twice. Add corn. Let stand covered for 10 minutes.

Yield: 10 servings of approximately 1 cup each. Freezes and/or reheats well.

179 calories per serving, 3 g fat (0.4 g saturated), 0 mg cholesterol, 9 g protein, 32 g carbohydrate, 431 mg sodium, 619 mg potassium, 4 mg iron, 9 g fiber, 81 mg calcium.

Notes and Variations:

- *A 19 oz (540 ml) can of beans or chickpeas contains 2 cups. Rinse well to remove excess sodium.*
- ***Gluten-Free Chili:*** *If you're allergic to wheat, do not use bulgur or couscous. Instead, substitute 1 cup of quinoa. Rinse thoroughly and drain well. Add to remaining ingredients and cook as directed.*
- *Serve over rice or noodles. Also great with Greek Salad (see page 100).*

Eggplant Roll-Ups

Eggplant replaces pasta in this simple and delicious vegetarian dish. Great for brunch!

1 medium eggplant (do not peel)
10 oz pkg (300 g) frozen spinach, cooked, drained and squeezed dry
1 cup pressed dry non-fat cottage cheese
3 tbsp grated Parmesan cheese
2 tbsp fresh basil, minced (or 1 tsp dried)
¼ cup skim milk
salt, pepper and garlic powder, to taste
2 cups tomato sauce
¾ cup grated low-fat mozzarella cheese

1. Preheat oven to 350°F. Slice eggplant lengthwise into 12 slices, discarding the outer slices. Arrange on a sprayed baking sheet. Bake for 10 minutes, until soft and pliable. Meanwhile, process spinach, cheeses, basil, milk and seasonings. Mix well. Pour 1 cup of sauce into a sprayed 9 x 13-inch casserole. Spread filling in a thin layer on each slice of eggplant and roll up tightly. Place seam side down in casserole. Top with remaining sauce and sprinkle lightly with cheese. Bake uncovered for 25 to 30 minutes, until golden and bubbling. Perfect with a garden salad.

Yield: 8 rolls. Freezes and/or reheats well. Double the recipe if you have guests.

102 calories per roll, 2.7 g fat (1.6 g saturated), 11 mg cholesterol, 10 g protein, 11 g carbohydrate, 582 mg sodium, 480 mg potassium, 1 mg iron, 3 g fiber, 173 mg calcium.

Enchilada Lasagna

No-roll enchiladas are layered like lasagna. Full of fiber and so calci-yummy!

2 tsp olive oil
1 onion, chopped
1½ cups mushrooms, sliced
1 green pepper, chopped
2 cloves garlic, crushed
3 cups tomato sauce (low-sodium, if possible)
19 oz (540 ml) can kidney beans (rinsed and drained)
½ tsp chili powder (to taste)
7 flour tortillas
¾ cup grated low-fat mozzarella cheese
¾ cup grated low-fat Swiss cheese

1. Preheat oven to 350°F. Heat oil in a non-stick skillet. Sauté veggies and garlic for 5 minutes. Add sauce, beans and chili powder. Simmer uncovered for 5 minutes. Spray a 2-quart casserole with non-stick spray. Layer 2 tortillas, ⅓ of sauce mixture and ⅓ of cheeses, until all ingredients are used, making 3 layers. Cut up the extra tortilla to fill in any empty spaces. Bake uncovered for 25 minutes.

Yield: 6 servings. Reheats and/or freezes well.

273 calories per serving, 5.8 g fat (2.2 g saturated), 13 mg cholesterol, 17 g protein, 41 g carbohydrate, 154 mg sodium, 617 mg potassium, 2 mg iron, 11 g fiber, 288 mg calcium.

Italian-Style Baked Tofu

1 lb firm tofu (500 g), sliced ½" thick (low-fat tofu can be used)
2 large onions, sliced
1 cup mushrooms, sliced
½ of a red pepper, chopped
½ of a green pepper, chopped
2½ cups vegetarian spaghetti sauce

1. Place sliced tofu between layers of paper towels on a plate. Top with another plate. Weigh it down with cans and let drain for 20 minutes. Preheat oven to 400°F. Spray a 9 x 13-inch casserole with non-stick spray. Place vegetables in the bottom of the dish. Add half of sauce and mix well. Place tofu on top of vegetable mixture. Top with remaining sauce. Bake uncovered for 40 to 45 minutes, basting once or twice during cooking.

Yield: 6 servings. Serve over pasta. Reheats well. Do not freeze.

213 calories per serving, 10.7 g fat (1.6 g saturated), 0 mg cholesterol, 15 g protein, 20 g carbohydrate, 560 mg sodium, 771 mg potassium, 10 mg iron, 5 g fiber, 192 mg calcium.

Pita Pizzas

So quick, so easy, so nutritious! Ideal as an appetizer, or perfect for kids as a quick meal. Pizzas can be topped with tuna, spinach, broccoli, cauliflower, zucchini, Parmesan cheese ... have it your way!

2–4 whole-wheat or white pitas (6½")
½ cup tomato sauce
6 sun-dried tomatoes, rehydrated and cut into strips (or 4 fresh tomatoes, sliced)
½ cup sliced red or green pepper

½ cup sliced mushrooms
¼ cup sliced onion, optional
2 tbsp fresh basil, minced (or ½ tsp dried)
1 cup low-fat grated mozzarella cheese

1. If pitas are thick, split them in half. Place cut-side up on a foil-lined baking sheet. Spread each pita with 2 tablespoons sauce. Add toppings. Bake in a preheated 425°F oven for 10 minutes, or until cheese melts and pizzas are piping hot. As appetizers, cut into 24 wedges with scissors or a pizza wheel.

Yield: 4 pizzas as a main dish or 24 wedges as an appetizer. These freeze and/or reheat well.

189 calories per pizza, 5.9 g fat (3.2 g saturated), 15 mg cholesterol, 12 g protein, 24 g carbohydrate, 576 mg sodium, 372 mg potassium, 2 mg iron, 4 g fiber, 223 mg calcium.

Notes:
- *To rehydrate sun-dried tomatoes: Cover tomatoes with boiling water. Let stand for 10 minutes. (Or cover with cold water and microwave on HIGH for 1 minute. Soak for 5 minutes, until soft.) Drain well. Scissors work well to cut up sun-dried tomatoes.*
- *For homemade sun-dried tomatoes, see page 285.*
- *As appetizers, each wedge contains 32 calories, 1 g fat (0.5 g saturated) and 3 mg cholesterol.*

Variations:
- ***Salsa Pita Pizzas:*** *Substitute salsa for tomato sauce. If desired, add 2 cloves of thinly sliced garlic. Monterey Jack can be used instead of mozzarella. Bake as directed. Cut into wedges.*

- ***Pesto Pita Pizzas:*** *Place pitas on a foil-lined pan. Spread each pita with 1 or 2 tablespoons Best-O Pesto (see page 149) or Sun-Dried Tomato Pesto (see page 163). Top with roasted red pepper strips. Allow half of a pepper per pizza. Sprinkle each pita with ¼ cup grated low-fat mozzarella. Bake in a preheated 425°F oven for 10 minutes, until cheese melts. Cut into wedges.*
- ***Tortilla Pizzas:*** *In any of the above pizzas, substitute three 9-inch flour tortillas for pitas. Before adding toppings to tortillas, pierce in several places with a fork to prevent them from puffing up. Bake directly on the oven rack in a preheated 400°F oven about 5 minutes, until crisp. Transfer to a foil-lined baking sheet and top with desired toppings. Sprinkle with grated cheese. (Salsa and Monterey Jack cheese are great!) Place under the broiler for a few minutes, until cheese melts. Cut into wedges.*

WELL-DRESSED PIZZAS

You can make your own pizzas in about the same time it takes to run out and buy one! These are all low in fat. Just be light-handed with the cheese and choose cheeses that are low fat or partly skimmed.

- Cheese, Tomato and Fresh Basil: Tomato sauce, fresh basil, grated mozzarella, sliced tomatoes and/or sun-dried tomatoes.
- Roasted Vegetable: Tomato sauce, oven-roasted or grilled vegetables (e.g., red peppers, roasted garlic, eggplant strips, sliced red onions, zucchini), grated Parmesan.
- Mediterranean: Sliced tomatoes, fresh or dried basil, crushed garlic, roasted red peppers, sliced black olives, grated Parmesan.
- Sun-Dried Tomato: Sun-dried tomatoes, fresh basil, garlic slivers, roasted red peppers, sliced green onions, tomatoes, grated Swiss or mozzarella.
- Dream Team Favorite: Tomato sauce, roasted red peppers, sun-dried tomatoes, sliced tomatoes, onions, sliced garlic, exotic mushrooms, fresh basil and grated mozzarella cheese.

- Mushroom and Spinach: Shiitake, porcini, portobello and/or cultivated mushrooms, chopped spinach, crushed garlic, roasted red peppers, red onions, grated mozzarella and/or Parmesan.
- Greek: Tomato sauce, sliced tomatoes, crumbled feta, chopped fresh spinach, black olives, green and red peppers, sliced onions, oregano, grated mozzarella.
- Artichoke and Spinach: Crushed garlic, olive oil, sliced artichoke hearts, chopped spinach, sliced mushrooms and tomatoes, grated mozzarella or cheddar.
- Ratatouille: Ratatouille (see below) and grated mozzarella or Swiss.
- Mexican: Salsa (homemade or bottled), sliced mushrooms, grated mozzarella or Monterey Jack.
- Chef's Secret: Use Quick 'n Easy Tomato Sauce (see page 159) or store-bought sauce. Buy low-sodium products if you're sodium-conscious (e.g., tomato or pizza sauce, tomato purée, tomato paste, canned tomatoes).
- Homemade Sun-Dried Tomatoes (see page 285) are wonderful on pizza, and simple to make! Prepare them in the fall, when tomatoes are plentiful, beautiful and inexpensive. (Rehydrate before using.)
- Sun-dried tomatoes packed in oil need to be rinsed very well before using to remove excess oil. Drain well and cut in strips with scissors.
- Roasted red peppers in a jar are very convenient to use, but they also need thorough rinsing to remove excess sodium.

Simple and Good Ratatouille (Mediterranean Vegetable Stew)

2 medium eggplants (2½ lb/1.2 kg)
2 medium onions
1 green and 1 red pepper
1 medium zucchini
2 cups mushrooms

4 cloves garlic, minced
1–2 tbsp olive oil
salt and pepper, to taste
½ tsp each dried basil and oregano
¼ cup balsamic or red wine vinegar
2 tbsp brown sugar (to taste)
2-5½ oz (156 ml) cans tomato paste
½ cup water

1. Spray a large, heavy-bottomed pot with non-stick spray. Dice vegetables (do not peel eggplant). Add oil to pot and heat on medium heat. Add vegetables and sauté for 10 to 15 minutes, stirring often. If necessary, add a little water to prevent sticking.
2. Add seasonings, vinegar, brown sugar, tomato paste and water. Simmer covered for 25 to 30 minutes, stirring occasionally. If mixture gets too thick, add a little water. Adjust seasonings to taste. Serve hot or cold.

Yield: 8 to 10 servings. Mixture keeps up to 10 days in the refrigerator or freezes well.

134 calories per serving, 2.4 g fat (0.4 g saturated), 0 mg cholesterol, 4 g protein, 28 g carbohydrate, 318 mg sodium, 906 mg potassium, 2 mg iron, 6 g fiber, 44 mg calcium.

Notes and Variations:

- *Delicious over spaghetti squash, rice, bulgur, couscous or your favorite grain.*
- *Ratatouille makes a great vegetarian pasta sauce. Serve it hot over spiral pasta or penne and sprinkle with grated low-fat mozzarella or Parmesan cheese. Heat for 2 minutes in the microwave to melt the cheese.*
- *Use Ratatouille instead of tomato sauce in lasagna. It also makes a great filling for crêpes. Leftover Ratatouille makes a perfect pizza topping.*
- *Serve a scoop of chilled Ratatouille on a bed of salad greens as a starter or light main course.*

177

- *Serve it cold as an appetizer with pita, low GI crackers or assorted breads.*
- ***Easy Vegetarian Stew:*** *In Step 2, add any of the following cut-up vegetables: yellow squash, celery, carrots, sweet potatoes, fresh or sun-dried tomatoes, green beans, asparagus. You can also add canned chickpeas, black beans and/or kidney beans, rinsed and drained. If desired, dice ½ pound (250 grams) of tofu and add to stew mixture during the last 10 minutes of cooking. (Tofu that was frozen, then thawed, will have a meaty texture.) Serve over rice, bulgur, pasta, or couscous.*

Spaghetti Squash "Noodle" Pudding

Spaghetti squash pulls into strands like spaghetti noodles, yet it has its own unique flavor. This recipe will have your guests guessing as to what the mysterious ingredient is! Although this recipe contains matzo meal, it is very well counteracted in terms of GI by lots of soluble fiber from the vegetables; and protein from the eggs, making it a low GI dish!

3 lb (1.2 kg) spaghetti squash (approximately)
2 onions, chopped
2 cloves garlic, crushed
1 tbsp olive oil
1 medium zucchini, finely grated
2 medium carrots, finely grated
2 eggs plus 4 egg whites (or 4 eggs)
½ cup matzo meal (found under Jewish or ethnic foods in your supermarket)
2 tbsp chopped fresh basil (or 1 tsp dried)
salt and pepper, to taste

1. Cut squash in half. Place cut-side down on a sprayed foil-lined pan. Bake at 350°F about 45 minutes, until tender. (Alternately, do not cut squash in half. Pierce it in several places with a fork. Microwave on HIGH until tender, 15 to 18 minutes, turning it over at half time. Let stand 15 minutes. Cut in half and let cool.)

178

2. Preheat oven to 375°F. In a non-stick skillet, sauté onions and garlic in oil for 5 minutes. Add zucchini and carrots and cook on medium heat until tender-crisp, about 5 minutes longer, stirring often. If necessary, add a little water to prevent burning or sticking. Cool slightly.

3. Discard squash seeds. Use a fork to pull out strands of squash. In a large mixing bowl, combine squash with remaining ingredients; season to taste. Transfer mixture to a sprayed 2-quart rectangular or oval casserole. Bake at 375°F for 50 to 60 minutes, until golden.

Yield: 10 to 12 servings. Reheats well.

101 calories per serving, 2.8 g fat (0.6 g saturated), 42 mg cholesterol, 5 g protein, 15 g carbohydrate, 87 mg sodium, 269 mg potassium, <1 mg iron, 3 g fiber, 43 mg calcium.

Note:
- *This recipe can be baked in sprayed individual ramekins or muffin pans. Bake at 375°F for 25 to 30 minutes, until golden.*
- *Delicious served as a dairy dish with non-fat yogurt.*
- *Cooked spaghetti squash is excellent served as an alternative to pasta. Top the strands of spaghetti squash with your favorite recipe of ratatouille or tomato sauce.*

Spinach Vegetable Pudding (a.k.a. Kugel)

The vegetables for this colorful, vitamin-packed kugel can be prepared quickly in the food processor. Double the recipe for a large crowd. It's a winner! Use frozen spinach instead of fresh if you prefer.

10 oz pkg (300 g) fresh spinach
2 onions, chopped
1 stalk celery, chopped
1 red pepper, chopped
3 carrots, grated

1 cup mushrooms, chopped
1 tbsp olive oil
2 eggs plus 2 whites (or 3 eggs)
¾ tsp salt
¼ tsp each pepper and garlic powder
½ tsp dried basil
¼ cup matzo meal (found under Jewish or ethnic foods in your
supermarket)

1. Preheat oven to 350°F. Wash spinach thoroughly. Remove and discard
    tough stems. Cook spinach in a covered saucepan until wilted, about 3
    minutes (or microwave on HIGH for 4 minutes). Don't add any water.
    The water clinging to the leaves will provide enough steam to cook it.
    Cool and squeeze dry.
2. Heat oil in a non-stick skillet on medium heat. Sauté onions, celery, red
    pepper and carrots for 5 minutes, until golden. Add mushrooms and
    cook 5 minutes longer. (Or cook vegetables uncovered in the microwave
    for 6 to 8 minutes on HIGH.)
3. Chop spinach coarsely. Combine with remaining ingredients and mix
    well. Pour into a sprayed 7 x 11-inch Pyrex casserole. Bake uncovered at
    350°F for 45 to 50 minutes, until firm. Cut in squares to serve.

Yield: 10 to 12 servings. Reheats well or may be frozen.

*81 calories per serving, 2.7 g fat (0.5 g saturated), 42 mg cholesterol, 4 g protein,
11 g carbohydrate, 241 mg sodium, 257 mg potassium, 2 mg iron, 2 g fiber,
52 mg calcium.*

Variation:

- ***Spinach Muffins:*** *Follow recipe above, but spoon batter into 12 sprayed
  muffin cups. Bake at 350°F for about 25 minutes, until golden. Serve as a
  side dish with meat, poultry or fish. Great for the lunch box!*

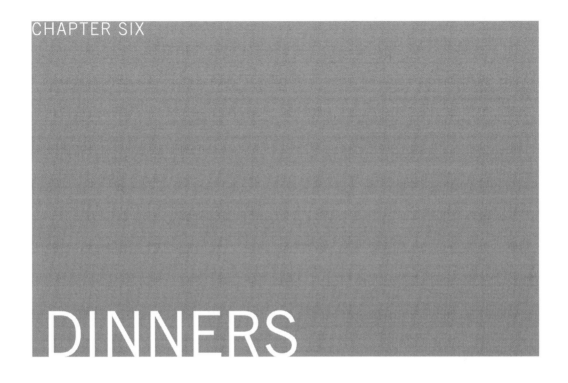

CHAPTER SIX

DINNERS

■ SOUPS

Bean, Barley and Sweet Potato Soup
(See recipe, page 82.)

Black Bean Soup
Excellent, easy and full of fiber! Impress your guests with its wonderful South American flavor.

 2 cups dried black beans, rinsed and drained
 6 cups cold water (for soaking the beans)
 2 onions, coarsely chopped
 4 cloves garlic, minced
 4 stalks celery, coarsely chopped
 1 tbsp olive oil
 4 large carrots, coarsely chopped
 1 tsp dried basil
 ½ tsp dried red pepper flakes
 1 tsp cumin (to taste)
 8 cups chicken or vegetable broth (about)
 salt and pepper, to taste

1. Soak beans overnight in cold water. Drain and rinse well. Discard soaking water.
2. Prepare vegetables. (This can be done in the processor.) Heat oil in a large soup pot. Add onions, garlic and celery. Sauté for 5 or 6 minutes on medium heat, until golden. If necessary, add a little water or broth to prevent sticking.
3. Add drained beans, carrots, seasonings and broth. Do not add salt and pepper until beans are cooked. Cover partially and simmer until beans are tender, about 2 hours, stirring occasionally. Purée part or all of the soup, if desired. If too thick, thin with water or broth. Add salt and pepper to taste.

Yield: 10 servings. Freezes well.

188 calories per serving, 2.1 g fat (0.3 g saturated), 0 mg cholesterol, 14 g protein, 29 g carbohydrate, 171 mg sodium, 495 mg potassium, 4 mg iron, 10 g fiber, 69 mg calcium.

Notes:

- *Soak and drain beans as directed in Step 1. Place soaked beans in a storage container and pop them in the freezer for up to 2 months. When you want to make soup, just add the frozen beans to the pot. No need to defrost them first. (You can use this trick with any kind of beans!)*
- *If you have time, presoak a batch of black beans, then cook them for 1½ to 2 hours, until tender. Drain, cool and freeze. When you want soup, add 3 to 4 cups of frozen cooked beans to the soup pot without thawing. Your soup will be ready in just half an hour!*
- *If you're really in a rush, substitute two 14 ounce (398 milliliter) cans of black beans, drained and rinsed, instead of soaking dried beans overnight. Cooking time with canned beans is also half an hour.*
- *Are you afraid to eat beans because you're worried about possible embarrassing moments? If you presoak beans, then discard the soaking water, you'll also eliminate the problem of gas! As an extra precaution, rinse the beans again thoroughly after presoaking them.*
- *Serving Tip: For an elegant touch, garnish each serving with a swirl of nonfat yogurt. If necessary, thin yogurt with a little milk. Use a plastic squeeze bottle to squeeze a design with the yogurt. Top with a spoonful of bottled or homemade salsa or chopped Roasted Red Peppers (see page 286).*

Greek-Style Lentil Soup

(See recipe, page 84.)

Green Split Pea and Barley Soup

(See recipe, page 85.)

Red Lentil, Vegetable and Barley Soup
(See recipe, page 87.)

Red Lentil, Zucchini and Couscous Soup
(See recipe, page 88.)

The Best Chicken Soup
(See recipe, page 90.)

Vegetable Broth ("Almost Chicken Soup")
(See recipe, page 92.)

■ SALADS AND DRESSINGS

Balsamic Salad Splash
(See recipe, page 93.)

Barley Salad with Honey Mustard Dressing
(See recipe, page 93.)

Creamy Cole Slaw
(See recipe, page 94.)

Creamy Cucumber Salad
(See recipe, page 95.)

Doug's "Flower Power" Caesar Salad
(See recipe, page 96.)

Easy Lentil Salad
(See recipe, page 97.)

Fattouche Salad
(See recipe, page 98.)

Fennel, Orange and Spinach Salad
(See recipe, page 99.)

Greek Salad
(See recipe, page 100.)

Greek-Style Black Bean Salad
(See recipe, page 101.)

Honey Mustard Carrot Salad
(See recipe, page 102.)

Honey Mustard Dressing
(See recipe, page 103.)

Israeli Salad
(See recipe, page 103.)

Jodi's Famous Bean Salad
(See recipe, page 104.)

Lighter Caesar Salad Dressing
(See recipe, page 105.)

Orange Balsamic Vinaigrette
(See recipe, page 106.)

Oriental Cole Slaw
(See recipe, page 107.)

Oriental Cucumber Salad
(See recipe, page 107.)

Quinoa Mandarin Salad
(See recipe, page 110.)

Rainbow Tabbouleh Salad
(See recipe, page 111.)

Ranch-Style Dressing
(See recipe, page 112.)

Red Cabbage Cole Slaw
(See recipe, page 113.)

Shake It Up Salad Dressing
(See recipe, page 114.)

Simply Basic Vinaigrette
(See recipe, page 115.)

Spinach and Mushroom Salad with Honey Mustard Dressing
(See recipe, page 116.)

Thousand Island Dressing (or Dip)
(See recipe, page 117.)

Tomato, Onion and Pepper Salad
(See recipe, page 119.)

■ SIDE DISHES

Barley and Mushroom Risotto

Pearl barley is more delicate in flavor than hulled (pot) barley, which is chewier and requires longer cooking. Barley is an excellent source of fiber. One cup of barley yields 3 cups cooked.

> 1 tbsp olive or canola oil
> 1 large onion, chopped
> 1 red pepper, chopped
> 2–3 cloves garlic, crushed
> 1½ cups mushrooms, sliced
> 1½ cups pearl barley, rinsed and well drained
> 3½ cups hot chicken or vegetable broth
> salt and pepper, to taste
> ¼ cup fresh dill, minced

1. In a large non-stick skillet, heat oil. Sauté onion, red pepper, garlic and mushrooms until golden, 5 to 7 minutes. Stir in barley and cook until lightly toasted, about 5 minutes. Slowly stir in ½ cup of hot broth. Cook, stirring, until it evaporates. Stir in another ½ cup broth. Repeat until you have added about 2 cups of broth. Pour in the remaining broth, cover and simmer for 45 minutes, until tender. If necessary, add a little water or broth to prevent sticking. Add salt, pepper and dill.

Yield: 8 servings. Reheats well or can be frozen. Leftovers can be used as a filling for Vegetarian Stuffed Peppers (see page 245).

177 calories per serving, 2.2 g fat (0.3 g saturated), 0 mg cholesterol, 7 g protein, 33 g carbohydrate, 79 mg sodium, 199 mg potassium, 2 mg iron, 7 g fiber, 28 mg calcium.

Beans and Carrots Amandine

Full of fiber and flavor. Yellow beans can be substituted. Almonds are a terrific source of calcium.

1 tsp tub margarine, butter or olive oil
2 cloves garlic, crushed
¼ cup sliced almonds
2 cups green beans, cut in half crosswise
2 cups carrots, cut into matchsticks
½ cup water
¼ tsp salt
½ tsp dried basil (or 1 tbsp fresh basil)
salt and pepper, to taste
2 tbsp grated Parmesan cheese, optional

1. Combine margarine and garlic in a 1 cup Pyrex measuring cup. Microwave uncovered on HIGH for 45 seconds. Stir in almonds. Microwave on HIGH for 3 to 4 minutes, until golden, stirring at half time. (Alternately, toast almonds with margarine and garlic in a non-stick skillet for 3 or 4 minutes.)
2. Combine green beans, carrots, water and salt in a 2-quart microsafe casserole. Microwave covered on HIGH for 7 to 8 minutes, stirring at half time. Let stand covered for 2 or 3 minutes. Veggies should be tender-crisp. Drain well. Combine vegetables with seasonings and almonds. Sprinkle with Parmesan cheese if desired.

Yield: 4 servings. Reheats well in the microwave.

120 calories per serving, 5.8 g fat (0.2 g saturated), 0 mg cholesterol, 4 g protein, 15 g carbohydrate, 207 mg sodium, 403 mg potassium, 2 mg iron, 6 g fiber, 79 mg calcium.

Broccoli, Mushroom and Pepper Sauté

This is great over pasta! Don't overcook broccoli, as heat destroys some of its protective antioxidants.

> 2 cups broccoli florets
> 4 cups cold water plus 1 tbsp vinegar
> 2 tsp olive oil
> 2 cloves garlic, crushed
> 2 cups mushrooms, sliced
> ½ cup red or yellow pepper, diced
> salt and pepper, to taste
> 1 tbsp fresh basil, minced (or ½ tsp dried)

1. Soak broccoli in cold water and vinegar for 10 minutes. Drain and rinse well. Steam broccoli for 2 to 3 minutes (or microwave it). In a large non-stick skillet, heat oil. Add garlic, mushrooms and pepper; stir-fry for 2 minutes. Add broccoli and stir-fry 2 minutes more. Add seasonings and serve.

Yield: 4 to 6 servings.

54 calories per serving, 2.7 g fat (0.4 g saturated), 0 mg cholesterol, 3 g protein, 7 g carbohydrate, 22 mg sodium, 368 mg potassium, 1 mg iron, 3 g fiber, 44 mg calcium.

Variations:

- ***Cauliflower, Mushroom and Pepper Sauté:*** Substitute cauliflower florets in the above recipe.
- ***Quick Basil and Orange Broccoli Sauté:*** Cover and microwave 3 cups cut-up broccoli on HIGH for 5 minutes. Add 2 tablespoons orange juice, 1 teaspoon margarine or olive oil, salt, pepper and a dash of basil. Yummy!

Carrot "Noodles"

6 medium carrots, peeled and trimmed
salt and pepper, to taste
½ tsp dried basil and/or dill
1 tsp olive oil or butter

1. With a carrot peeler, use long strokes to make thin parings that look like noodles. Boil carrots 3 to 4 minutes, until almost tender; drain well. Mix with seasonings and olive oil. Serve immediately.

Yield: 4 servings. Do not freeze.

55 calories per serving, 1.3 g fat (0.2 g saturated), 0 mg cholesterol, 1 g protein, 11 g carbohydrate, 66 mg sodium, 232 mg potassium, <1 mg iron, 3 g fiber, 35 mg calcium.

Couscous and Mushroom Casserole

Many people think that couscous is a grain, but it's actually a pasta made from hard durum wheat. The bran and germ are stripped from the wheat berry, then the endosperm (semolina) is ground, steamed and dried to form tiny grains. There is also a delicious whole-wheat couscous available, with its natural bran layers intact.

1 cup couscous
2 cups water, chicken or vegetable broth
6 green onions, chopped
1 red and/or green pepper, chopped
3 cloves garlic, minced
2 tsp olive or canola oil
1 cup mushrooms, sliced
1 cup canned chickpeas or black-eyed peas, drained and well-rinsed

1 medium carrot, grated
salt and pepper, to taste
½ tsp dried basil
2 tbsp minced fresh dill (or 1 tsp dried)

- *Microwave Method:* Combine couscous and water or broth in a 2-quart microsafe casserole and let stand. (Water will be absorbed by the couscous.) Combine green onions, peppers, garlic and oil in a microsafe bowl. Microwave uncovered on HIGH 3 to 4 minutes, until softened. Stir in mushrooms and cook 2 minutes longer. Add to couscous along with chickpeas, carrot and seasonings. Microwave covered on HIGH for 5 minutes, or until remaining liquid is absorbed. Fluff with a fork to separate the grains. Adjust seasonings to taste.
- *Conventional Method:* In a large saucepan or skillet, sauté green onions, peppers and garlic in oil until softened. Add mushrooms and sauté 3 to 4 minutes longer. Add water or broth and bring to a boil. Stir in couscous along with remaining ingredients. Bring back to a boil, cover and simmer until all the liquid is absorbed, about 5 to 10 minutes. Fluff with a fork to separate the grains. Adjust seasonings to taste. (If mixture seems dry, add a little extra liquid.)

Yield: 6 servings of approximately ¾ cup each. Freezes and/or reheats well.

196 calories per serving, 2.3 g fat (0.3 g saturated), 0 mg cholesterol, 7 g protein, 37 g carbohydrate, 155 mg sodium, 251 mg potassium, 2 mg iron, 5 g fiber, 42 mg calcium.

Variations:

- **Couscous Middle-Eastern Style:** *Omit basil and dill. Replace with ½ teaspoon each of ground cumin, ginger and cinnamon. If desired, cook ¼ cup currants or raisins along with the couscous. For a delicious, crunchy texture, stir ¼ cup toasted pine nuts into couscous just before serving.*

191

- ***Couscous American-Style:*** *Cook ⅓ cup dried cranberries (craisins) along with couscous. Stir ¼ cup toasted, chopped pecans into cooked couscous just before serving.*
- ***Couscous Italian-Style:*** *Add 1 cup diced zucchini and 1 cup canned diced tomatoes (with juice) to sautéed vegetables. Cook 5 minutes longer. Stir in couscous along with remaining ingredients. Omit dill and add 2 tablespoons fresh minced basil. (Chickpeas can be omitted, if desired.)*

Fruit and Vegetable "Stew" (a.k.a. Tsimmis)

In Yiddish, a tsimmis means much ado about nothing. This colorful, vitamin-packed stew is really something! It's not only full of fiber, beta carotene and potassium, it tastes terrific.

¾ cup pitted prunes
¾ cup dried apricots
⅓–½ cup raisins
2 lb (1 kg) carrots, peeled and sliced
1 sweet potato, peeled, quartered and sliced
½ cup honey (to taste)
14 oz (398 ml) can pineapple chunks, drained (reserve ½ cup juice)
½ cup orange juice
salt and pepper, to taste
2 tsp pareve tub margarine
1 tsp cinnamon

1. Soak prunes, apricots and raisins in boiling water to cover for ½ hour, until plump. Drain well. Meanwhile, cook carrots and sweet potato in boiling water until tender but firm, about 15 minutes. Drain well. Combine reserved pineapple juice with remaining ingredients except pineapple chunks; mix gently. Place mixture in a sprayed 3-quart casserole. Bake covered in a preheated 350°F oven for 35 minutes. Stir in pineapple chunks and bake uncovered 15 minutes more, basting once or twice.

Yield: 10 servings. Freezes and/or reheats well.

195 calories per serving, 1.1 g fat (0.2 g saturated), 0 mg cholesterol, 2 g protein, 48 g carbohydrate, 66 mg sodium, 581 mg potassium, 2 mg iron, 6 g fiber, 52 mg calcium.

Glazed Apricot Carrots with Peppers

> 2 lb carrots, peeled and sliced
> 1 red pepper, diced
> 1 onion, diced
> ¼ cup apricot jam (preferably low-sugar)
> 2 tbsp fresh dill, minced
> salt and pepper, to taste

1. Slice carrots ½-inch thick. Cook in boiling salted water until nearly tender, about 10 to 12 minutes. Add red pepper and onion and simmer 4 or 5 minutes longer. Drain well and return to heat. Stir in jam and dill; mix well. Add salt and pepper to taste.

Yield: 6 servings.

100 calories per serving, 0.4 g fat (0.1 g saturated), 0 mg cholesterol, 2 g protein, 24 g carbohydrate, 96 mg sodium, 381 mg potassium, 1 mg iron, 5 g fiber, 50 mg calcium.

Glazed Sweet Potatoes

Sweet potatoes are virtually fat-free and provide nearly half the recommended daily nutrient intake of vitamin C. Most important of all, they're delicious!

> 2 onions, peeled and sliced
> 4 sweet potatoes, peeled and cut in 2" chunks
> 2 tsp olive oil or melted margarine

2 tbsp maple syrup or honey
salt and pepper, to taste
¼ tsp dried basil
¼ cup orange juice

1. Preheat oven to 375°F. Spray a 2-quart covered Pyrex casserole with non-stick spray. Arrange onions in the bottom of the casserole; add sweet potatoes. Drizzle with olive oil and maple syrup. Sprinkle with seasonings. Drizzle orange juice over potatoes. Rub sweet potatoes well to coat them evenly with mixture. Cover and bake at 375°F for 45 minutes. Uncover and bake 15 minutes longer, stirring once or twice, until potatoes are tender and golden.

Yield: 6 servings. Reheats well, but do not freeze.

158 calories per serving, 1.9 g fat (0.3 g saturated), 0 mg cholesterol, 2 g protein, 34 g carbohydrate, 15 mg sodium, 278 mg potassium, <1 mg iron, 3 g fiber, 36 mg calcium.

Note:
- *Time-Saving Secret! Microwave potatoes covered on HIGH for 12 to 14 minutes, stirring once or twice, they will be partially cooked. Transfer casserole to a preheated 375°F oven. Bake uncovered 20 to 25 minutes, until tender, basting occasionally. If necessary, add a little more orange juice or water to casserole.*

Grilled Skewered Vegetables

These are a great vegetable dish for your next BBQ. Miniature vegetables are a nice alternative. They are often available at specialty produce stores.

1 Japanese or small eggplant, cut in 1" chunks
salt, to taste
12-4" wooden skewers

2 red peppers, cut in 1" chunks

2 medium zucchini, sliced ½" thick

2 green peppers, cut into 1" chunks

1 large or 2 medium onions, cut into 1" chunks

12 cherry tomatoes

½ cup bottled fat-free or low-calorie Italian salad dressing

2 tbsp minced fresh basil and/or parsley

1. Sprinkle eggplant with salt. Place on a baking sheet and cover with another baking sheet. Weigh down with several cans; let drain 20 minutes. Rinse well; pat dry. Soak wooden skewers in cold water for 20 minutes. Arrange veggies alternately on skewers, starting with eggplant, then red pepper, zucchini, green pepper, onion and cherry tomato. Drizzle with salad dressing and marinate for 20 to 30 minutes. (Skewers can be prepared in advance up to this point and marinated for several hours.)

2. Preheat grill or broiler. Grill or broil vegetables about 4 inches from heat until nicely browned, about 3 to 4 minutes per side. Sprinkle with basil and/or parsley. Serve hot or at room temperature.

Yield: 12 kabobs. Allow 2 per person. Freezing is not recommended.

28 calories per kabob, 0.2 g fat (0 g saturated), 0 mg cholesterol, 1 g protein, 6g carbohydrate, 100 mg sodium, 216 mg potassium, trace iron, 1 g fiber, 11 mg calcium.

High-Fiber Turkey Stuffing

1–2 tbsp olive oil

2 onions, chopped

3 stalks celery, chopped

2 cups mushrooms, sliced

3 carrots, grated

10 slices of low GI rye or multi-grain bread
2 apples, cored, peeled and chopped
salt and pepper, to taste
2 tbsp fresh dill, chopped
2 tbsp fresh basil, chopped (or 1 tsp dried)
1 tbsp fresh thyme (or 1 tsp dried)
½–¾ cup chicken broth

1. Heat oil in a large, non-stick skillet. Sauté onions and celery until golden. Add mushrooms and carrots. Cook 5 minutes longer; remove from heat. Cut bread into cubes and add to skillet with remaining ingredients. Mix well. You will have enough for a 10 to 12-pound turkey. (Stuffing can be prepared up to 24 hours in advance and refrigerated, but don't add broth until just before cooking.) Remove excess fat from turkey neck and cavity. Stuff turkey loosely. Fold neck skin over and attach it with a skewer to the turkey. Cook turkey as per recipe directions, allowing 25 to 30 minutes per pound.

Yield: 10 servings. Reheats well. Freezing not recommended.

132 calories per serving, 2.6 g fat (0.7 g saturated), 0 mg cholesterol, 4 g protein, 24 g carbohydrate, 245 mg sodium, 182 mg potassium, 2 mg iron, 3 g fiber, 43 mg calcium.

Variations:
- ***Skinnier Stuffing:*** *Bake stuffing separately in a covered greased casserole at 325°F for 1 hour.*
- ***Stuffin' Muffins:*** *Bake stuffing in sprayed muffin tins at 350°F for 25 minutes, until crispy.*

Homemade Baked Beans

Full of flavor, fiber, iron and calcium, yet low in fat. These are a nutritional bargain. No time to make beans? For a great shortcut, add 2 to 3 tablespoons maple syrup to a can of baked beans. Just heat and eat!

1 lb (454 g) white beans (e.g., navy)
6 cups water
2 onions, chopped
¼ cup sugar (white or brown)
⅓ cup molasses
2 tbsp red wine vinegar
1¾–2 cups tomato juice
1 tsp dry mustard
¼ tsp cayenne (to taste)
½ tsp black pepper
salt, to taste

1. Soak beans overnight; rinse and drain well. Cook in 6 cups unsalted water for 45 to 60 minutes, until tender. Reserve cooking water from beans; set aside. Preheat oven to 275°F. In an ovenproof dish, combine drained beans with remaining ingredients plus 1 cup of reserved cooking water. Bake covered until tender, about 5 hours. Add more water if needed to prevent mixture from drying out.

Yield: 10 servings. These taste even better a day or two later!

215 calories per serving, 0.8 g fat (0.2 g saturated), 0 mg cholesterol, 10 g protein, 44 g carbohydrate, 160 mg sodium, 674 mg potassium, 4 mg iron, 7 g fiber, 105 mg calcium.

Kasha and Bow Ties with Mushrooms.

(See recipe, page 153.)

Lentil and Rice Casserole (Medjaderah)

A Middle-Eastern favorite. Uli Zamir makes this vegetarian dish at least once

a week. 1 cup brown lentils, rinsed and drained

6 cups water, divided

1 tbsp canola oil

2 onions, chopped

3–4 cloves garlic, minced

salt and pepper, to taste

1 tbsp pareve soup mix (chicken flavor)

1 tsp ground cumin (or to taste)

1½ cups long-grain rice

¼ cup coriander (cilantro), chopped

1. Bring lentils and 3 cups of water to a boil. Reduce heat and cook covered for 15 minutes, until partially cooked. Drain well. Meanwhile, heat oil in a non-stick skillet. Sauté onions and garlic in oil until golden, about 5 minutes. Add salt, pepper, soup mix and cumin. Cook until well browned, about 10 minutes, stirring often. Add rice, drained lentils and remaining 3 cups of water. Cover and simmer 20 to 25 minutes, until rice is tender. Add more water if necessary during cooking. Stir in coriander and adjust seasonings to taste. For a terrific vegetarian meal, serve with Israeli Salad (see page 103).

Yield: 10 servings. Reheats well. Freezing is not recommended.

198 calories per serving, 2.1 g fat (0.2 g saturated), trace cholesterol, 7 g protein, 37 g carbohydrate, 214 mg sodium, 266 mg potassium, 3 mg iron, 5 g fiber, 36 mg calcium.

Marinated Mushrooms

Absolutely addictive! Serve warm or cold. These are also excellent as an appetizer or a salad.

> 2 lb mushrooms
> 1 tbsp olive oil
> ½ of a small onion, finely chopped
> 4–5 large cloves garlic, minced
> ¾ cup dry white wine
> juice of half a lemon
> ¼ cup chicken or vegetable broth
> ¼ tsp dried rosemary, crushed
> ¼ tsp dried thyme
> salt and pepper, to taste
> ¼ cup fresh parsley, chopped
> 1 tbsp minced fresh dill, if desired

1. Rinse mushrooms quickly and pat dry with paper towels. If mushrooms are large, cut them in half or in thick slices.
2. In a large non-stick skillet, heat olive oil on medium heat. Add onion and sauté for about 5 minutes, until tender. Add mushrooms and garlic. Sauté on medium heat until mushrooms begin to release their juices, about 6 to 8 minutes. Stir often. Add wine, lemon juice, broth, seasonings, parsley and dill. Bring to a boil and reduce heat. Simmer uncovered, stirring occasionally, for about 20 minutes, or until mushrooms are tender. Adjust seasonings to taste. If desired, garnish with additional parsley.

Yield: about 8 servings of ½ cup each. These keep for 2 or 3 days in the refrigerator. Do not freeze.

49 calories per serving, 1 g fat (trace saturated), 0 mg cholesterol, 2 g protein, 6 g carbohydrate, 51 mg sodium, 345 mg potassium, 2 mg iron, 2 g fiber, 15 mg calcium.

199

Note:

- *Chef's Trick! An egg slicer is great for slicing mushrooms (and kiwis too)!*

Minted Peas with Red Peppers

Green peas are more nutritious than green beans! They contain vitamins A and C and are high in fiber.

> 10 oz pkg (300 g) frozen green peas
> 2 tsp tub margarine or olive oil
> 4 green onions (white part only), chopped
> 1 red pepper, chopped
> 1–2 tbsp fresh mint, minced
> salt and freshly ground pepper, to taste
> 1 tbsp fresh lime or lemon juice

1. Bring a saucepan of water to a boil. Add peas and simmer 3 to 4 minutes, until tender-crisp. Drain and rinse well under cold water to stop the cooking process. Set aside. Melt margarine in a non-stick skillet. Add onions and red pepper. Sauté for 4 or 5 minutes, until softened. Add peas and mint. Cook for 1 to 2 minutes, just until heated through. Add seasonings and lime juice. Serve immediately.

Yield: 3 to 4 servings.

104 calories per serving, 2.8 g fat (0.5 g saturated), 0 mg cholesterol, 5 g protein, 16 g carbohydrate, 99 mg sodium, 217 mg potassium, 2 mg iron, 5 g fiber, 29 mg calcium.

Variation:

- ***Rice Pea-laf with Peppers:*** *Prepare Minted Peas with Red Peppers as directed above. Combine with 3 cups of cooked brown basmati rice. Add salt and pepper to taste.*

Oven Roasted Vegetables (Ratatouille-Style)

These vegetables are scrumptious served hot over pasta, at room temperature over salad greens, or at any temperature as a side dish. Any way you serve them, they're a winner!

1 medium eggplant, cut in strips or slices
1 tsp salt
1 large red onion, halved and sliced
2 red peppers, cut in strips or slices
2 green peppers, cut in strips or slices
2 medium zucchini, cut in strips or slices
1 cup mushrooms, sliced
4 tomatoes, sliced
4 cloves garlic, crushed
2 tbsp olive oil
2 tbsp lemon juice or rice wine vinegar
2 tsp dried basil (or 2 tbsp fresh, minced)
½ tsp dried thyme, if desired
salt and pepper, to taste

1. Sprinkle eggplant strips or slices with salt. Place in a colander or strainer over a bowl. Let stand 20 minutes. Press out excess liquid. Combine with remaining ingredients in a large mixing bowl and mix well. (May be prepared 3 or 4 hours in advance, covered and refrigerated until needed.) Spread in a single layer on a large baking sheet that has been sprayed with non-stick spray.
2. Preheat oven to 450°F. Bake uncovered on top rack of oven for 20 to 25 minutes, or until well browned and tender-crisp. Stir 2 or 3 times during cooking.

Yield: 8 servings. Reheats well, especially in the microwave. Do not freeze.

97 calories per serving, 4 g fat (0.6 g saturated), 0 mg cholesterol, 2 g protein, 16 g carbohydrate, 303 mg sodium, 562 mg potassium, 1 mg iron, 4 g fiber, 32 mg calcium.

Variation:

- ***Barbecued Vegetables:*** *Slice eggplant and onions ½-inch thick. Seed and core peppers; cut in quarters. Trim ends off zucchini, cut in half or thirds crosswise, then slice lengthwise. Use large mushrooms, but grill just the caps. (Portobellos are excellent.) Omit tomatoes. Preheat the grill. Rub vegetables with garlic, olive oil, lemon juice and seasonings. Place veggies in a sprayed perforated grill pan or basket. Grill for 6 to 8 minutes per side, until browned and tender-crisp. An alternative is to wrap veggies in heavy-duty foil packets (one per person), seal tightly and grill for 20 to 30 minutes.*

Note:

- *Time- and Fat-Saving Secret! Instead of rubbing the veggies with garlic, oil, lemon juice and seasonings, substitute bottled fat-free Italian salad dressing.*

Quick and Simple Zucchini

4 medium zucchini, sliced ¼" thick
salt and pepper, to taste
1 tbsp fresh lemon or lime juice
2 tbsp fresh basil, chopped (or 1 tsp dried)
2 tsp soft margarine

1. Place zucchini slices in a round microsafe casserole. Sprinkle with seasonings and lemon juice. Cover and microwave on HIGH for 5 minutes, until tender-crisp, stirring at half time. Let stand for 1 to 2 minutes. Stir in margarine. Serve immediately.

Yield: 4 servings. Reheats well in the microwave.

38 calories per serving, 2 g fat (0.3 g saturated), 0 mg cholesterol, <1 g protein, 5 g carbohydrate, 20 mg sodium, 322 mg potassium, <1 mg iron, 2 g fiber, 19 mg calcium.

Variation:

- **Quick Stewed Zucchini:** *Slice 2 pounds of zucchini. Heat 1 tablespoon olive oil in a non-stick skillet. Sauté zucchini in oil until golden, about 6 to 8 minutes, stirring often. Add 2 cloves of crushed garlic and cook 2 minutes longer. Add a 19-ounce can (540 ml) tomatoes (with juice), 1 teaspoon sugar and ½ teaspoon dried basil. Cover and simmer for 15 to 20 minutes, stirring occasionally. Makes 6 servings.*

Quinoa

Quinoa (keen-wah) was the staple food of the Incas for more than 5,000 years. An excellent source of iron, magnesium and potassium, it contains complex carbohydrates and high quality protein. Quinoa provides lysine, an amino acid missing from corn and wheat, and is very easy to digest. It's available at natural food shops. Store it in the fridge or freezer; it will keep for 3 to 4 months.

> 2 cups water, vegetable or chicken broth
> 1 cup quinoa
> 1 clove garlic
> pinch of salt

1. Bring water or broth to a boil. Place quinoa in a fine-meshed strainer. Rinse under running water to remove the bitter coating (saponin). Rinse until water runs clear; drain well. Add quinoa, garlic and salt to boiling liquid. Reduce heat and simmer covered for 15 minutes. Don't overcook. Remove from heat and let stand covered for 5 minutes. Fluff with a fork. If any liquid remains, drain in a strainer. Use quinoa instead of rice in pilafs, or in grain-based salads.

Yield: About 3 cups (6 servings).

107 calories per serving, 1.7 g fat (0.3 g saturated), 0 mg cholesterol, 4 g protein, 20 g carbohydrate, 57 mg sodium, 212 mg potassium, 3 mg iron, 2 g fiber, 20 mg calcium.

Variation:
- ***Crimson Quinoa:*** *Add 1 cup canned grated beets, well-drained, to hot quinoa. Mix well. Add 4 minced green onions, 2 tablespoons raspberry or balsamic vinegar, 1 tablespoon lemon juice and 2 tablespoons extra-virgin olive oil. Season with salt and pepper. Serve at room temperature.*

Rainbow Rice Pilaf

Colorful and vitamin-packed, this easy side dish also makes a fabulous filling for Vegetarian Stuffed Peppers (see page 245). Fresh vegetables can be used instead of frozen.

2 cups vegetable broth
1 cup long-grain or basmati rice, rinsed and drained
2 tsp olive oil
1 large onion, finely chopped
2 cloves garlic, crushed
½ cup green pepper, finely chopped
½ cup red pepper, finely chopped
1 cup zucchini, finely chopped
1½ cups frozen mixed vegetables, thawed
salt and pepper, to taste
½ tsp dried basil

1. In a medium saucepan, bring broth to a boil. Add drained rice to saucepan, cover and simmer on low heat for 20 minutes. Remove from heat and let stand covered for 10 minutes. Meanwhile, heat oil in a non-stick skillet. Add onion and sauté for 5 minutes. Add garlic, peppers and zucchini. Sauté 4 or 5 minutes longer, until tender-crisp. If necessary, add

a little broth or water to prevent sticking. Stir in mixed vegetables. Cover and let stand for 5 minutes to heat through. Combine veggie mixture with rice. Season to taste. Fluff with a fork.

Yield: 6 servings. Leftovers keep 2 days in the fridge and reheat well. Freezing is not recommended.

193 calories per serving, 2.3 g fat (0.3 g saturated), 0 mg cholesterol, 6 g protein, 39 g carbohydrate, 355 mg sodium, 238 mg potassium, 2 mg iron, 4 g fiber, 36 mg calcium.

Roasted Onions

These are an excellent substitute for sautéed onions. So sweet, and no added fat! Roasted onions can be stored in the refrigerator for 2 or 3 days in a tightly closed container. I don't bother freezing them because they cook so quickly in the microwave. Onions are a natural decongestant. They may help lower blood pressure and cholesterol and may help decrease the ability of the blood to clot.

- *Micro-Roasted Onions:* (Ideal when you need only 1 or 2 sautéed onions.) Rinse onions, then pierce in several places with a sharp knife. Don't bother peeling them! Place on a plate and microwave on HIGH for 3 to 4 minutes for 1 onion, 6 to 7 minutes for 2 onions. To test for doneness, insert a sharp knife; onions should be very tender. Cooking time depends on size. When cool, peel and chop.
- *Oven-Roasted Onions:* (Ideal when you need a large amount of sautéed onions.) Rinse onions but do not peel. Pierce in several places with a sharp knife. Place on a sprayed baking sheet and bake in a preheated 400°F oven for 45 to 50 minutes, until tender. When cool, peel and chop.

57 calories per large onion, 0.2 g fat (0 g saturated), 0 mg cholesterol, 2 g protein, 13 g carbohydrate, 4 mg sodium, 213 mg potassium, trace iron, 2 g fiber, 28 mg calcium.

205

Ruthie's Oven-Grilled Veggies with Basil

Ruthie Dressler is an energetic, spiritual, beautiful lady who cooks the most tantalizing vegetarian dishes. The high oven temperature creates a scrumptious, grilled taste.

    4 ripe, firm tomatoes
    2 large sweet onions (e.g., Spanish)
    3–4 colored peppers (red, green, yellow and/or orange)
    3–4 zucchini (about 1 lb/500 g)
    2 tbsp olive oil
    coarse salt, to taste
    ¼ cup fresh basil, chopped

1.   Preheat oven to 500°F. Cut tomatoes in wedges. Slice onions, peppers and zucchini into long strips. Place veggies on a foil-lined baking sheet. Drizzle with olive oil and sprinkle with coarse salt. Bake uncovered for 15 minutes, until slightly blackened and tender. Add basil and mix well. This tastes somewhat like a grilled ratatouille and is great hot or cold.

Yield: 6 to 8 servings. Do not freeze. Serve with pasta, rice, millet or bulgur.

119 calories per serving, 5.2 g fat (0.7 g saturated), 0 mg cholesterol, 3 g protein, 18 g carbohydrate, 16 mg sodium, 645 mg potassium, 1 mg iron, 4 g fiber, 37 mg calcium.

Sesame Broccoli

    1 large bunch broccoli (1½ lb/750 g)
    2 tbsp sesame seeds
    1 tsp Oriental sesame oil
    1 tbsp fresh lemon juice
    1 tbsp brown sugar
    salt and pepper, to taste

1. Cut up broccoli, slicing stems thinly. Rinse well. Steam (or microwave covered on HIGH with 2 tablespoons water) for 5 to 7 minutes, until tender-crisp. Place sesame seeds in a small pan and toast on medium heat for 3 or 4 minutes. Watch carefully to prevent burning. Drain broccoli; combine with sesame oil, lemon juice, brown sugar and seasonings. Top with toasted sesame seeds.

Yield: 4 servings. Can be reheated briefly in the microwave.

97 calories per serving, 3.8 g fat (0.3 g saturated), 0 mg cholesterol, 6 g protein, 13 g carbohydrate, 56 mg sodium, 568 mg potassium, 2 mg iron, 6 g fiber, 99 mg calcium.

Variations:

- **Sesame Green Beans:** *Substitute one pound green beans. Steam (or microwave) for 6 to 7 minutes. Beans should be crisp and bright green. Drain and continue with recipe.*
- **Quick Cauliflower Crown:** *Trim leaves from cauliflower but leave it whole. Rinse and drain well. Place on a microsafe plate, cover it with an inverted glass bowl and microwave on HIGH for 7 to 8 minutes. Let stand covered for 3 minutes. Omit brown sugar. Season with salt, pepper and lemon juice. Top with sesame seeds.*

Simply Sautéed Greens

1 tbsp olive oil
1 red pepper, chopped
2–3 cloves garlic, crushed
2 lb greens, well-trimmed, washed and drained

1. In a wok or large skillet, sauté red pepper and garlic in oil for 2 minutes. Chop tender leaves into 1-inch pieces and add gradually to the pan. Reduce heat to medium, cover and cook until tender, stirring occasionally.

(Beet greens and spinach take 2 to 3 minutes, Swiss chard and broccoli rabe take 3 to 4 minutes, and kale takes 5 to 8 minutes.) Add a few tablespoons of water if mixture becomes dry. Season with salt and pepper. Remove greens from the pan with a slotted spoon.

Yield: 4 servings.

114 calories per serving (for kale), 4.4 g fat (0.6 saturated), 0 mg cholesterol, 5 g protein, 15 g carbohydrate, 54 mg sodium, 579 mg potassium, 2 mg iron, 3 g fiber, 176 mg calcium.

Simply Steamed Asparagus

1½ lb (750 g) asparagus, trimmed and cut into 2" slices
salt and pepper, to taste
1 tsp fresh thyme leaves (or ¼ tsp dried)
3 tbsp fresh lemon, lime or orange juice
1 tsp tub margarine (or 2 tsp light tub margarine)

1. Soak asparagus in cold water; drain well. Steam for 3 to 4 minutes. Immediately transfer to a bowl of ice water to stop the cooking process. (To microwave asparagus, place it in an oval casserole and microwave covered on HIGH for 6 to 7 minutes, until tender-crisp. Let stand covered for 3 minutes.) Season with salt, pepper and thyme. Sprinkle with juice. Add margarine and mix well. At serving time, reheat for 2 or 3 minutes on HIGH in the microwave.

Yield: 4 to 6 servings. Do not freeze.

50 calories per serving, 1.5 g fat (0.3 g saturated), 0 mg cholesterol, 4 g protein, 8 g carbohydrate, 26 mg sodium, 269 mg potassium, 1 mg iron, 3 g fiber, 35 mg calcium.

Variations:
- ***Asparagus Vinaigrette:*** *Steam asparagus as directed. Omit lemon juice and margarine. Sprinkle asparagus with salt, pepper and thyme. Toss with non-fat or low-fat Italian salad dressing or Honey Mustard Dressing (see page 103).*

Spaghetti Squash "Noodle" Pudding
(See recipe, page 178.)

Spinach Vegetable Pudding (a.k.a. Kugel)
(See recipe, page 179.)

Squished Squash
Nutrient-packed, rich in beta-carotene and folic acid, this dish is potassi-yummy!

2 acorn squash or 1 butternut squash
1–2 tbsp tub margarine or olive oil
salt and pepper, to taste
¼ tsp each of ground cinnamon and nutmeg

1. Preheat oven to 375°F. Cut squash in half crosswise. Place cut-side down on a sprayed non-stick baking pan. Bake uncovered until tender, about 50 to 60 minutes.
2. Cool slightly, then scoop out and discard seeds and stringy pulp from squash. Scoop out the flesh from squash into a bowl and mash together with margarine/olive oil and seasonings. Reheat before serving.

Yield: 4 servings. Do not freeze.

103 calories per serving, 3.1 g fat (0.6 g saturated), 0 mg cholesterol, 2 g protein, 20 g carbohydrate, 30 mg sodium, 601 mg potassium, 1 mg iron, 6 g fiber, 65 mg calcium.

Notes:
- *To microwave squash, pierce in several places with a sharp knife. Place on microsafe paper towels and microwave on HIGH, allowing 5 to 7 minutes per pound. Turn squash over halfway through cooking. Total cooking time will be 12 to 14 minutes. Complete as directed in Step 2.*
- *Squash anyone? Winter varieties include acorn, buttercup, butternut, Hubbard, pumpkin, spaghetti and turban squash. They do not need refrigeration. Store at room temperature for about a month.*

Stewed Cabbage or Brussels Sprouts with Noodles

Cabbage and Brussels sprouts may help prevent certain cancers. They're also rich in vitamin C.

> 1 tbsp olive or canola oil
> 2 onions, chopped
> 2 cloves garlic, crushed
> 3 cups finely sliced cabbage (or 1 lb Brussels sprouts, trimmed and cut in quarters)
> ½ of a red pepper, chopped
> 1 carrot, grated
> ¾ cup chicken or vegetable broth
> salt and pepper, to taste
> 2 cups cooked noodles (preferably yolk-free)

1. In a large non-stick skillet, heat oil. Add onions and sauté for 5 minutes. Add garlic, cabbage or sprouts, red pepper, carrot and broth. Cook uncovered for 6 to 7 minutes, stirring occasionally, until softened. Stir in seasonings and noodles. Cook just until heated through.

Yield: 6 to 8 servings.

171 calories per serving, 3.9 g fat (0.6 g saturated), trace cholesterol, 6 g protein, 29 g carbohydrate, 43 mg sodium, 204 mg potassium, 2 mg iron, 4 g fiber, 52 mg calcium.

Turkish Bulgur Pilaf

A gem of a recipe from Suzi Lipes of Montreal. She often prepares this colorful, nutrition-packed pilaf for dinner guests, hoping she'll have leftovers to enjoy the next morning for breakfast!

1½ cups Spanish onion, chopped
3 stalks celery, chopped
1 red pepper, chopped
1 tbsp olive oil
½ cup fresh dill, minced
2 cups bulgur, rinsed and drained
2½ cups boiling chicken or vegetable stock
½ cup raisins or currants, rinsed and drained
1 cup dried apricots, rinsed and chopped
½ tsp salt (to taste)
¼ cup chopped toasted nuts, if desired
½ cup fresh parsley, minced

1. In a large skillet, sauté onions, celery and red pepper in hot oil on medium-high heat for 5 to 7 minutes, until golden. Add dill and bulgur. Cook uncovered 4 or 5 minutes longer, stirring often.
2. Carefully pour in boiling liquid. Add raisins, apricots and salt. Cover and simmer for 20 minutes, until liquid is absorbed. Remove from heat and let stand for 5 minutes. Stir in nuts and parsley and fluff with a fork. Serve hot.

Yield: 10 to 12 servings. Reheats and/or freezes well. Leftovers keep for 4 or 5 days in the fridge.

175 calories per serving, 1.9 g fat (0.3 g saturated), 0 mg cholesterol, 6 g protein, 36 g carbohydrate, 180 mg sodium, 402 mg potassium, 2 mg iron, 7 g fiber, 38 mg calcium.

Notes:

- *Slivered almonds, pecans or pine nuts are delicious in this dish. Almonds are high in calcium. With almonds, one serving of pilaf contains 196 calories, 3.6 grams fat (0.4 saturated) and 47 milligrams calcium.*
- *Toasting brings out the full flavor of nuts, so a little flavor goes a long way. Toast nuts uncovered for 8 to 10 minutes at 350°F. It's okay to enjoy a little decadence on special occasions!*
- *You can also substitute millet or quinoa instead of bulgur.*
- *How to toast bulgur, millet and other grains: Rinse and drain well. Place in a large heavy-bottomed skillet. Toast on medium heat for about 5 minutes, stirring constantly to prevent burning. (It's ready when it gives off a toasty aroma and makes a light popping sound.) Remove pan from heat. Add liquid slowly to prevent spattering. Add vegetables and seasonings. Cover and simmer until done, about 20 minutes. Remove from heat and let stand covered for 10 minutes.*

Vegetable Platter Primavera

2 cups broccoli florets
2 cups cauliflower florets
1 cup carrots, sliced on the bias
1 cup sliced zucchini or yellow squash
4 green onions (white part only), sliced
½ cup red pepper, diced
1 tbsp olive oil (or melted margarine)
2 tbsp lemon juice
1 tbsp water
salt and pepper, to taste
2 tbsp minced fresh basil and/or dill

1. Soak broccoli, cauliflower and carrots in cold water for 10 minutes. Drain well but do not dry. Arrange broccoli and cauliflower florets in a ring around the outer edge of a large microwave-safe plate. Make an inner ring of carrots, then of zucchini. Place green onions and red pepper in the centre. Combine olive oil, lemon juice and water; drizzle over vegetables. Cover with an inverted Pyrex pie plate or a damp paper towel.
2. Microwave covered on HIGH for 6 to 8 minutes, until tender-crisp. Let stand covered for 2 minutes. Season with salt, pepper and herbs. Serve immediately.

Yield: 6 servings. Do not freeze.

62 calories per serving, 2.7 g fat (0.4 g saturated), 0 mg cholesterol, 3 g protein, 9 g carbohydrate, 111 mg sodium, 351 mg potassium, <1 mg iron, 4 g fiber, 45 mg calcium.

Vegetarian Harvest Oven Stir-Fry
So colorful, so healthy!

1 medium eggplant, unpeeled
1 red, 1 yellow and 1 green pepper
1 medium Spanish onion (about 2 cups)
2 medium zucchini, unpeeled
2 cups sliced mushrooms (try shiitake or portobello)
4 cloves garlic, crushed
1 tbsp olive oil
2 tbsp balsamic or red wine vinegar
salt and pepper, to taste
2 tbsp fresh chopped rosemary or basil (or 1 tsp dried)

1. Preheat oven to 425°F. Cut eggplant, peppers, onion and zucchini into narrow strips. Combine all ingredients in a large bowl. (May be prepared in advance, covered and refrigerated for 3 or 4 hours.) Spread in a thin

layer on a large foil-lined baking sheet that has been sprayed with
non-stick spray.

2. Place baking sheet on top rack of oven. Bake uncovered for 25 to 30
    minutes, until tender-crisp and lightly browned, stirring once or twice.

Yield: 6 servings. This dish reheats well either in the microwave or conventional
oven. Veggies become soggy if frozen.

*99 calories per serving, 3 g fat (0.4 g saturated), 0 mg cholesterol, 3 g protein, 18 g
carbohydrate, 8 mg sodium, 532 mg potassium, 2 mg iron, 5 g fiber, 55 mg calcium.*

■ FISH DISHES

The following dishes may be served with Basmati, brown or long grain rice.

Baked Halibut Parmesan

4 halibut steaks (1½ lb/750 g)
salt, pepper and dried basil, to taste
2 cloves garlic, crushed (or ½ tsp garlic powder)
2–3 tbsp fat-free or light mayonnaise (or yogurt)
4 tsp grated Parmesan cheese
paprika, to garnish

1. Preheat oven to 450°F. Arrange fish in a single layer on a non-stick or
    sprayed baking sheet. Sprinkle lightly with seasonings. Brush the top
    side of fish with mayonnaise. Sprinkle with cheese and paprika.
    Bake uncovered at 450°F for 10 to 12 minutes, until golden. Serve
    immediately.

Yield: 4 servings. Do not freeze.

185 calories per serving, 4.2 g fat (0.9 g saturated), 51 mg cholesterol, 33 g protein, 2 g carbohydrate, 174 mg sodium, 702 mg potassium, 1 mg iron, 0 g fiber, 103 mg calcium.

Notes and Variations:

- *Also excellent with sea bass, salmon, rainbow trout, salmon trout, sole or orange roughy fillets. Bake uncovered at 450°F, allowing 10 minutes per inch of thickness for fish.*
- ***Rosy Halibut:*** *Add 1 tablespoon Sun-Dried Tomato Pesto (see page 163) to mayonnaise or yogurt; use to coat fish. You can also use a mixture of equal parts of puréed roasted red peppers and yogurt.*
- ***Baked Fish with Tahini:*** *Combine 4 tablespoons tahini, 6 tablespoons water, 2 cloves garlic and a dash of fresh lemon juice. Sprinkle fish with salt and pepper. Coat fish on both sides with tahini mixture; sprinkle with paprika. Bake at 450°F for 10 to 12 minutes, until golden.*

Baked Herbed Fish Fillets

(See recipe, page 132.)

Easy Pesto Fish Fillets

(See recipe, page 133.)

Gloria's Sea Bass with Honey Mustard

4 sea bass steaks (about 1½ lb/750 g)
2 tsp olive oil
2 tbsp prepared honey-style mustard
2 cloves garlic, minced
2 tbsp fresh lemon juice
2 tbsp chopped parsley
salt and pepper, to taste

1. Preheat oven to 450°F. Rinse fish; pat dry. In a small bowl, combine oil, mustard, garlic, lemon juice and parsley. Season fish with salt and pepper; coat with mustard mixture. Place on a sprayed foil-lined pan. Bake at 450°F, allowing 10 minutes cooking time per inch of thickness, about 10 to 12 minutes. If overcooked, fish will be dry.

Yield: 4 servings. Serve flaked leftover fish over mixed salad greens.

187 calories per serving, 5.5 g fat (1.1 g saturated), 61 mg cholesterol, 27 g protein, 6 g carbohydrate, 196 mg sodium, 411 mg potassium, <1 mg iron, trace fiber, 26 mg calcium.

Variation:
- **Quick Sea Bass with Balsamic Marinade:** *Coat fish with Orange Balsamic Vinaigrette (see page 106) or bottled low-fat balsamic salad dressing. Bake uncovered at 450°F for 10 to 12 minutes.*

Grilled Moroccan Salmon
If broiling fish in your oven, spray broiler rack with non-stick spray to prevent sticking.

4 salmon fillets or steaks (1.5 lb/750 g)
1 tsp ground cumin
½ tsp paprika
1 tsp thyme
salt and pepper, to taste
½ tbsp olive oil
1 tbsp fresh lemon juice
1 lemon, sliced

1. Preheat grill or broiler. Sprinkle both sides of salmon with seasonings. Drizzle lightly with olive oil and lemon juice. If using the grill, place fish in a lightly greased grill basket. Grill over hot coals (or under the broiler) 3 to 4 minutes per side. Grill lemon slices quickly. Use as a garnish for salmon.

Yield: 4 servings.

333 calories per serving, 15.7 g fat (2.4 g saturated), 121 mg cholesterol, 44 g protein, 2 g carbohydrate, 97 mg sodium, 1109 mg potassium, 2 mg iron, <1 g fiber, 38 mg calcium.

Micropoached Salmon Fillets
(See recipe, page 134.)

Quick Pickled Salmon
(See recipe, page 137.)

Salmon Balsamico
Tuna steaks are also delicious prepared this way. Serve with pasta or vegetables.

> 4 pieces salmon fillets (1½ lb/750 g)
> salt and freshly ground pepper, to taste
> ¼ cup balsamic vinegar
> 2 tsp brown sugar
> 2 cloves garlic, crushed
> 2 Italian (Roma) tomatoes, chopped
> 1–2 tbsp chopped fresh basil or 1 tsp dried (1 tsp thyme can be substituted)

1. Arrange fish in a single layer in a sprayed baking dish. Sprinkle lightly with salt and pepper. Combine vinegar with brown sugar, garlic, tomatoes and basil; pour over fish. Marinate for 30 minutes. Preheat oven to 450°F. Bake uncovered for 10 to 12 minutes. (To microwave fish, cover with a layer of lettuce leaves or a piece of cooking parchment. Cook on HIGH for 6 to 8 minutes, or until fish flakes with a fork. If you wet the parchment, you can mold it around the dish.)

Yield: 4 servings. Delicious hot or cold.

285 calories per serving, 13 g fat (2.3 g saturated), 102 mg cholesterol, 33 g protein, 7 g carbohydrate, 85 mg sodium, 535 mg potassium, 1 mg iron, <1 g fiber, 25 mg calcium.

Variations:

- ***Sea Bass or Tuna Balsamico:*** *Substitute sea bass or tuna steaks for salmon. One serving of bass contains 205 calories, 4.3 grams fat (1 gram saturated), 144 milligrams cholesterol and 553 milligrams potassium.*

Sea Bass Thai Style
You'll be hooked on this fish dish! Delicate and delectable.

> 4 portions of sea bass (1½ lb/750 g)
> 2 green onions
> 2 tbsp coriander (cilantro) and/or basil leaves
> 1 slice ginger (1 to 2 tsp minced)
> 2 cloves garlic
> salt and pepper, to taste
> ¼ tsp cayenne
> 1 tsp Oriental sesame oil

1. Spray a foil-lined baking sheet with non-stick spray. Place fish on baking sheet. Mince green onions, coriander, ginger and garlic. (I use the processor.) Rub mixture on both sides of fish. Season with salt, pepper and cayenne; brush with sesame oil. Let stand at room temperature for 20 minutes, or cover and refrigerate for up to 2 hours. Preheat oven to 450°F. Bake fish uncovered for 10 to 12 minutes, until golden. Fish should flake when lightly pressed. Serve immediately.

Yield: 4 servings. Leftover fish can be broken into chunks and served on chilled salad greens.

157 calories per serving, 4 g fat (1 g saturated), 61 mg cholesterol, 27 g protein, 1 g carbohydrate, 101 mg sodium, 405 mg potassium, <1 mg iron, trace fiber, 23 mg calcium.

Sesame Salmon

Open the "weigh" to a healthy heart! Serve with basmati rice and steamed green and yellow beans.

> 4 pieces salmon fillets (about 1½ lb/750 g)
> juice of ½ a lemon (or 1 tbsp rice vinegar)
> 2 tbsp lite soy sauce
> 1 tbsp maple syrup or honey
> 1 tsp Oriental sesame oil
> 2 cloves garlic, crushed
> 1 tbsp grated ginger
> paprika
> 1 tbsp sesame seeds

1. Place salmon in a baking dish that has been sprayed with non-stick spray. Sprinkle salmon with lemon juice. Combine remaining ingredients except sesame seeds and rub over salmon. Let marinate for 20 to 30 minutes. Meanwhile, preheat oven to 425°F. Sprinkle salmon lightly with sesame seeds. Bake uncovered for 12 to 15 minutes (or microwave covered on HIGH for 6 to 8 minutes), until fish flakes when lightly pressed.

Yield: 4 servings. Leftovers can be broken into chunks and added to salad greens or pasta.

284 calories per serving, 13.2 g fat (1.9 g saturated), 94 mg cholesterol, 34 g protein, 4 g carbohydrate, 529 mg sodium, 856 mg potassium, 2 mg iron, trace fiber, 32 mg calcium.

Note:

- *Chef's Secret! When microwaving fish, place it between wet lettuce leaves; this prevents fish from popping during cooking. Parchment paper also makes an excellent cover. Place parchment under running water. It will become flexible so you can mold it around the baking dish easily!*

Tuna Caponata
(See recipe, page 138.)

Tuna, Rice and Broccoli Pudding
(See recipe, page 140.)

■ CHICKEN AND TURKEY

The following dishes may be served with Basmati, brown or long grain rice.

SLIM CHICK-INFORMATION

- Go for the white and you'll be light; discard the skin and you'll be thin!
- Compare the white meat from a quarter of a chicken (skinless breast, without the wing) to the dark meat (skinless drumstick and thigh). White meat has 3.1 grams fat, dark meat has 8.2 grams fat.
- One roasted single chicken breast, with skin, has 193 calories, 7.6 grams fat (2.2 grams saturated) and 82 milligrams cholesterol. Remove the skin and it will have 142 calories, 3.1 grams fat (0.9 grams saturated) and 73 milligrams cholesterol.
- One roasted drumstick, with skin, has 112 calories, 5.8 grams fat (1.6 grams saturated) and 47 milligrams cholesterol. Without skin, it has 76 calories, 2.5 grams fat (0.6 grams saturated) and 41 milligrams cholesterol.
- One roasted thigh, with skin, has 154 calories, 9.6 grams fat (2.7 grams saturated) and 58 milligrams cholesterol. Without skin, it has 109 calories, 5.7 grams fat (1.6 grams saturated) and 50 milligrams cholesterol.

- Did you know that 1 roasted chicken wing with skin has 99 calories, 6.6 grams fat (1.9 grams saturated) and 29 milligrams cholesterol? It's difficult to remove the skin, so use wings in soup.

- A 3 pound (1.4 kilo) chicken (with skin) contains 1,547 calories, 88 grams fat (25 grams saturated) and 570 milligrams cholesterol. Remove the skin and the calories will fly away!

- Lighten up with turkey! A 3 ounce serving of roasted skinless turkey breast has 115 calories, 0.6 grams fat (0.2 grams saturated) and 71 milligrams cholesterol. The same amount of skinless dark meat has 159 calories, 6.1 grams fat (2.1 grams saturated) and 72 milligrams cholesterol.

- Ground chicken and turkey are often loaded with fat and contain dark meat, increasing the fat content. Know what you're eating! Ask your butcher to grind just the skinless breast meat for you, or grind it yourself quickly in the processor. Remove and discard the skin, bone and excess fat. Cut poultry breast into 1-inch chunks. Process for 15 to 20 seconds, until minced.

- Raw poultry can be frozen for about 6 months at 0°F if properly wrapped.

- Once raw poultry has thawed, it cannot be refrozen unless you cook it first. For example, if your freezer breaks down and your chicken has thawed, cook it. Then you can freeze it again.

- Never defrost poultry at room temperature. Either defrost it in the refrigerator overnight or use the microwave. It takes 5 to 6 minutes per pound (10 to 12 minutes per kilo) on DEFROST. Boneless breasts take 4 to 5 minutes per pound (3 or 4 single boneless breasts weigh about 1 pound.) Arrange thicker pieces outward and thinner pieces inward. Remember: thin is in!

- After defrosting poultry in the microwave, it should still be cold to the touch. The ice crystals in the thicker parts will dissolve shortly. Rinse in cold water and let stand 5 to 10 minutes before cooking. Cook immediately, or refrigerate once it is completely defrosted.

- Poultry, whether cooked or raw, should not be left on the counter for more than an hour during the summer, or for more than 2 hours during the winter, to prevent food poisoning.
- To prevent salmonella and cross-contamination, everything that touches raw poultry should be washed with a sanitizing solution of 1 tablespoon bleach dissolved in 1 gallon (4 liters/quarts) of warm (not hot) water. Let surfaces air dry; do not rinse. Discard leftover solution.
- Koshered chickens have already been salted, so don't sprinkle them with salt before cooking. Adjust seasonings at the end of cooking. To remove excess salt from Koshered chickens, soak them in several changes of cold water before cooking.
- Skin or no skin? If roasting poultry without a sauce, leave skin on during cooking to keep it moist; remove skin after cooking. If cooking poultry in sauce, remove skin before cooking. Otherwise, fat from the skin melts and drains into the sauce.

Cajun Chicken Breasts

Add a little spice to your life. Simply fantastic, and so versatile!

4 boneless, skinless chicken breasts
½ tbsp olive oil
2 tbsp lemon juice
 salt and freshly ground pepper (to taste)
½ tsp chili powder
½ tsp paprika
½ tsp cayenne
½ tsp dried basil
2 cloves garlic, crushed

1. Rinse chicken and pat dry. Trim off excess fat. Combine oil, lemon juice, seasonings and garlic in a mixing bowl. Add chicken and marinate for an

hour at room temperature, or up to 24 hours covered in the refrigerator. (Refer to "Fowl Play" in tips following this recipe.)

2. Preheat oven to 400°F. Remove chicken from marinade and arrange in a single layer on a foil-lined 10 x 15 x 1-inch baking sheet. Pour marinade over and around chicken. Bake uncovered for 20 minutes, turning chicken pieces over at half time. Baste occasionally with pan juices. When done, chicken will be springy when lightly touched. If overcooked, chicken will be tough.

Yield: 4 servings. Cooked chicken may be dry if frozen and reheated.

163 calories per breast, 4.9 g fat (1.1 g saturated), 73 mg cholesterol, 27 g protein, 2 g carbohydrate, 69 mg sodium, 257 mg potassium, 1 mg iron, trace fiber, 22 mg calcium.

Notes and Variations:

- *Fowl Play: Marinate a batch of chicken breasts, then freeze in meal-sized packages for up to a month. (Never do this with chicken that was previously frozen, then defrosted!) When needed, thaw chicken overnight in the refrigerator (or in the microwave) and then cook as directed.*
- *Leftovers? Make Lighter Chicken Salad (see page 142). Chilled leftover chicken can also be thinly sliced across the grain and used for sandwiches with low GI bread.*
- ***Cajun Chicken Tid-Bites:*** *These are yummy appetizers. Follow recipe for Cajun Chicken Breasts (above), but cut chicken into 1-inch pieces. (Each breast yields about 8 pieces.) Marinate and cook as directed, reducing cooking time to 15 minutes. Serve on toothpicks as hors d'oeuvres. Also great served on a bed of salad greens. Serve with salsa (bottled or homemade).*
- ***Grilled Cajun Chicken Breasts:*** *Preheat grill or broiler. Marinate chicken as directed. Remove from marinade and pat dry. Grill or broil over medium to medium-high heat about 5 to 7 minutes on each side. Baste chicken frequently with marinade; don't overcook. Cooking time on the grill will be shorter than under the broiler because of the higher, direct heat.*

- *BBQ Chip Tips: For a gourmet touch, soak 3 or 4 handfuls of wood chips (mesquite, applewood, hickory) in water for at least half an hour. Toss the soaked chips on top of the hot coals just before placing chicken on.*

Chicken Pepperonata

This scrumptious dish certainly doesn't taste like the usual chicken! It's sure to become a new family favorite.

12 boneless, skinless chicken breasts, trimmed of fat
pepper and paprika, to taste
2 tbsp olive or vegetable oil
3 tbsp lemon juice (juice of a lemon)
4 green peppers, cut into strips
2 red peppers, cut into strips
4 onions, sliced
28 oz can (796 ml) tomatoes, drained and chopped
5½ oz can (156 ml) tomato paste
½ cup sweet or dry red wine
3–4 cloves garlic, minced
2 tbsp sugar or honey (to taste)
1 tbsp additional lemon juice (to taste)
½ cup raisins, rinsed and drained (optional)

1. Place chicken breasts in a large bowl. Sprinkle lightly with seasonings. Add oil and lemon juice. Rub into chicken. Marinate chicken at least ½ hour at room temperature, or up to 24 hours in the refrigerator. (You can freeze the chicken at this point if it wasn't previously frozen. Defrost overnight in the refrigerator when needed.)
2. Preheat oven to 400°F. Spray 2 foil-lined baking sheets with non-stick spray. Arrange chicken in a single layer on 1 pan. Combine any leftover marinade with peppers and onions and spread them on the other pan. (If you're short of marinade, add a little more lemon juice to

the vegetables.) Bake uncovered at 400°F for 15 to 18 minutes, until chicken is just baked through and vegetables are softened, but still bright in color. Transfer chicken to a large shallow baking dish. Reserve vegetables.

3. Meanwhile, prepare sauce. Combine drained tomatoes, paste, wine, garlic, sugar and remaining lemon juice in a skillet. Simmer uncovered for 10 minutes; stir occasionally. Add raisins and simmer sauce 3 or 4 minutes longer.

4. Pour sauce over chicken. Reduce oven heat to 350°F. Bake covered for 15 minutes. Uncover, add vegetables and mix well. Bake covered 10 to 15 minutes longer.

Yield: 12 servings. Reheats and/or freezes well, but vegetables will be softer if frozen.

237 calories per serving, 5.6 g fat (1.2 g saturated), 73 mg cholesterol, 29 g protein, 16 g carbohydrate, 288 mg sodium, 646 mg potassium, 2 mg iron, 2 g fiber, 52 mg calcium.

Notes:
- *If desired, cut chicken into chunks or strips. This makes it easy to serve if you've made several main dishes. Your guests can taste a little bit of each dish without waste or guilt!*
- *For variety, add sliced zucchini and mushrooms to vegetable mixture in Step 2.*

Chicken with Bulgur and Mushrooms
Easy, tasty and nutritious!

3 lb (1.4 kg) chicken, cut in pieces
3 onions, sliced
2 cups mushrooms, sliced
1 cup bulgur, rinsed and well-drained

2 cloves garlic, minced
salt (optional)
freshly ground pepper, to taste
1 tsp dried basil
2 cups vegetarian tomato sauce
¾ cup water

1. Wash chicken and remove skin. Trim off excess visible fat. Place onions, mushrooms and bulgur in the bottom of a lightly greased casserole. Arrange chicken pieces on top. Rub chicken with garlic and seasonings. Combine sauce and water; pour over chicken and bulgur. Bake covered at 350°F for 1¼ hours, or until chicken is tender and most of liquid is absorbed. Adjust seasonings to taste.

Yield: 6 servings. Reheats and/or freezes well.

330 calories per serving, 10 g fat (2.3 g saturated), 72 mg cholesterol, 29 g protein, 33 g carbohydrate, 516 mg sodium, 851 mg potassium, 3 mg iron, 7 g fiber, 60 mg calcium.

Notes:
- *If desired, chicken wings can be set aside and frozen. When you have enough saved up, make chicken soup!*
- *Serve with steamed zucchini and carrots seasoned with salt, pepper and dill.*

Dracula Chicken
Spicy and luscious, this simple dish was a hit at our festive dinners!

2 chickens (about 3 lb/1.4 kg each)
2–3 tbsp coarse steak spices
1 tbsp paprika

1 tbsp dried basil
3 onions, sliced
¾–1 cup water

1. Trim fat from chicken. Rub chicken under the skin with seasonings. Arrange a bed of onions in the bottom of a sprayed roasting pan. Place chicken on top of onions. Cover and refrigerate overnight.
2. Preheat oven to 350°F. Add water to chicken. Cook covered 1½ hours, until tender. Uncover and cook ½ hour longer, until golden and crispy, basting occasionally. If necessary, add a little extra water to the pan. Let stand for 20 minutes. Cut up into serving-sized pieces, removing the skin to reduce fat. Strain fat from pan juices with a fat separator. Place pan juices in a gravy boat to serve.

Yield: 12 servings. Reheats and/or freezes well.

182 calories per serving, 6.7 g fat (1.8 g saturated), 72 mg cholesterol, 25 g protein, 5 g carbohydrate, 269 mg sodium, 320 mg potassium, 2 mg iron, 1 g fiber, 39 mg calcium.

Gloria's Limelight Roast Chicken

Gloria Schachter gave me this moist and luscious chicken recipe, which I've adapted. Yummy!

3½ lb (1.6 kg) whole chicken
salt and freshly ground pepper, to taste
1 tsp dried basil
3 limes
1–2 stalks celery, cut into chunks
¼ cup chopped parsley or coriander (cilantro)

227

1. Rinse chicken and dry well. Loosen skin; rub seasonings inside the cavity and under skin of chicken. Squeeze juice of 1 lime over chicken. Marinate for 1 hour at room temperature or cover and marinate in the fridge overnight. Pierce limes with a fork. Place limes, celery and parsley inside the chicken. Close up openings with metal skewers. Place chicken on its side in a roasting pan.

2. Preheat oven to 425°F. Roast uncovered for 20 minutes. Turn chicken onto its other side and roast 20 minutes more. Reduce heat to 350°F and roast breast-side up 20 minutes longer, until golden and crisp. Remove chicken from oven. Strain fat from pan juices. Place pan juices in a gravy boat. Cut up chicken; remove skin, limes, celery and parsley. Garnish with additional lime slices.

Yield: 6 servings. Reheats and/or freezes well. Recipe can be doubled for company.

191 calories per serving, 7.4 g fat (2 g saturated), 84 mg cholesterol, 28 g protein, 1 g carbohydrate, 92 mg sodium, 308 mg potassium, 2 mg iron, trace fiber, 26 mg calcium.

Herb Roasted Chicken

So flavorful, so moist! This recipe will become part of your regular repertoire.

3 lb (1.4 kg) chicken, cut into pieces
2–3 cloves garlic, crushed
½ tsp each of dried basil, oregano and rosemary
¼ tsp dried thyme
1 tsp Hungarian paprika
freshly ground pepper
1 tbsp olive oil

1. Wash chicken well and pat dry. Loosen chicken skin but don't remove it. Rub flesh of chicken with garlic, seasonings and olive oil. Cover chicken and marinate at least an hour (or preferably overnight) in the refrigerator to allow the flavor of the herbs to penetrate.
2. Preheat oven to 400°F. Place chicken pieces skin-side down on a rack in a foil-lined pan. Roast chicken uncovered for 15 minutes. Reduce heat to 350°F. Roast chicken skin-side up for 1 hour, or until golden and juices run clear. Baste occasionally. Remove skin before serving.

Yield: 6 servings. Recipe may be doubled or tripled, if desired. Freezes well.

183 calories per serving, 8.7 g fat (2.1 g saturated), 72 mg cholesterol, 24 g protein, trace carbohydrate, 72 mg sodium, 228 mg potassium, 1 mg iron, trace fiber, 17 mg calcium.

Notes and Variations:

- *Chef's Fat-Saving Secrets! Loosen the skin from breasts, legs and thighs of chicken. Rub garlic, seasonings and oil over chicken under the skin. Cook as directed; remove skin before serving. Skin keeps chicken moist and bastes it without adding extra fat. Discard fatty drippings before serving.*
- ***Shortcut BBQ Chicken:*** *Prepare chicken as directed in Step 1. Preheat the BBQ or grill. Place chicken in a Pyrex casserole and microwave covered on HIGH for 8 to 9 minutes. Turn chicken pieces over, moving small pieces to the center. Microwave 7 to 8 minutes longer. Transfer partly-cooked chicken to hot grill immediately. Cook 15 to 20 minutes longer, until crispy and golden. Remove skin before serving.*
- *Chef's BBQ Secrets! Chicken will be very juicy if microwaved before grilling. To prevent flare-ups, grill chicken over heat, not flame.*
- *Chicken is high in protein and an excellent source of phosphorus and nicacin. It's also a good source of iron, zinc and riboflavin.*

Herbed Lemon Chicken Breasts with Mushrooms

Elegant and luscious, yet so easy!

4 boneless, skinless chicken breasts, trimmed
¼ cup fresh lemon juice
1 tsp olive oil
salt and freshly ground pepper, to taste
1 tsp dried rosemary
1 tsp dried thyme
1 tbsp additional olive oil
2 cups shiitake or cremini (brown) mushrooms, sliced
3 large cloves garlic, thinly sliced
3 tbsp white wine or brandy
2 tbsp fresh parsley, minced

1. Butterfly each chicken breast by cutting it almost in half, then open it like a book to make a large, thin piece. Place in a single layer in a glass casserole. Sprinkle with lemon juice, oil and seasonings. Marinate covered in the refrigerator for several hours or overnight.

2. Heat oil in a large non-stick frypan. Add mushrooms and garlic. Season lightly with salt and pepper and sauté on medium-high heat about 5 minutes, until browned. Remove pan from heat and transfer mushrooms to a bowl.

3. Return pan to the heat and pour in marinade from chicken. Add chicken breasts to hot marinade and brown on medium-high heat for 3 to 4 minutes per side, until cooked through. Remove chicken from pan. Stir in wine or brandy and scrape up any browned bits from the bottom of the pan. Return chicken and mushrooms to pan and cook 2 or 3 minutes longer to heat through. Sprinkle with parsley. Serve immediately.

Yield: 4 servings. If reheating this dish, add a little chicken broth or water to create steam (about ¼ to ½ cup). This prevents it from drying out. Heat covered for a few minutes, just until piping hot.

241 calories per serving, 8 g fat (1.6 g saturated), 73 mg cholesterol, 28 g protein, 13 g carbohydrate, 69 mg sodium, 357 mg potassium, 2 mg iron, 2 g fiber, 34 mg calcium.

Jamaican Jerk Chicken

Chili peppers are very hot, so use rubber gloves when handling!

> 3½ lb chicken (1.6 kg), cut up
> 2 onions, cut in chunks
> 3 cloves garlic
> 2 tbsp ginger
> 1 hot chili pepper, cored and seeded
> ½ tsp ground allspice
> 1 tsp pepper
> 1 tsp dried thyme (or 1 tbsp fresh)
> 3 tbsp red or white wine vinegar
> 3 tbsp soy sauce

1. Rinse chicken; trim fat. Grind onions, garlic, ginger and chili pepper in the processor. Mix in remaining ingredients except chicken. Coat chicken with sauce. Cover and marinate overnight in the fridge. Place chicken on a rack in a foil-lined broiling pan. Place a pan of water in the bottom of the oven. Roast chicken uncovered at 375°F for 45 minutes, basting often. Preheat broiler or grill. Grill or broil chicken until crusty, about 15 minutes. Remove skin before serving.

Yield: 6 servings. Reheats and/or freezes well.

221 calories per serving, 7.6 g fat (2.1 g saturated), 84 mg cholesterol, 29 g protein, 7 g carbohydrate, 544 mg sodium, 376 mg potassium, 2 mg iron, 1 g fiber, 34 mg calcium.

Lemon Dill Chicken in a Pouch

This is a perfect dish for one person or for a crowd. For a large quantity, multiply all ingredients. Easy and versatile! Cold leftovers are delicious thinly sliced and served on a crusty roll or in a salad.

> 1 boneless, skinless chicken breast, trimmed of fat (¼ lb/125 g)
> salt, if desired
> freshly ground pepper, to taste
> paprika, to taste
> 1 tsp fresh dill, minced (or ½ tsp dried)
> ½ tsp olive or canola oil
> 1–2 tbsp fresh lemon juice

1. Place chicken in a bowl and sprinkle it with seasonings. Rub with dill, oil and lemon juice. Let marinate for 30 minutes at room temperature, or cover and refrigerate up to 24 hours.
2. Cut a large square of foil or parchment paper. Place chicken on the foil and drizzle lightly with marinade. Seal package by crimping edges closed. (If preparing several portions, make individual packages.) Place on a baking sheet and bake in a preheated 400°F oven for 20 to 25 minutes. (Use a toaster oven for 1 or 2 portions.) To serve, place pouch on a serving plate and cut open at the table.

Yield: 1 serving. Best served immediately, but if you make a large quantity, leftovers can be reheated. Cooked chicken might be too dry if frozen (see "Time-Saving Secret" below).

145 calories per serving, 4.9 g fat (1.1 g saturated), 63 mg cholesterol, 23 g protein, 1 g carbohydrate, 55 mg sodium, 209 mg potassium, <1 mg iron, trace fiber, 13 mg calcium.

Notes and Variations:

- *Perfect with steamed rice (see lower GI rice choices at the start of this section) and broccoli florets or a garden salad.*

- *Time-Saving Secret! Combine chicken with seasonings, dill, oil and lemon juice in an airtight container. Freeze for up to 1 month. Thaw overnight in the fridge, or use the microwave. (One piece of chicken takes 2 to 3 minutes on DEFROST.) Cook immediately as directed in Step 2.*

- *Forget-about-the-Pouch Version: Place marinated breasts on a lightly greased baking sheet. Bake uncovered at 400°F for 20 minutes.*

- ***Grilled or Broiled Lemon Chicken:*** *Preheat grill or broiler. Prepare chicken as directed in Step 1. Remove chicken from marinade and pat dry. Grill or broil over medium-high heat, allowing 5 to 6 minutes per side. Baste often with marinade. Do not overcook or chicken will be dry.*

- *Microwave Method: In Step 2, wrap marinated chicken breasts in parchment paper. Cook 3 minutes on HIGH for 1 single breast, 4 to 4½ minutes for 2 single breasts, and 6 to 7 minutes for 4 single breasts (1 to 1¼ pounds). When done, chicken juices should run clear.*

- ***Chicken and Vegetables in a Pouch:*** *Prepare Lemon Dill Chicken as directed, but before sealing package(s), top chicken with one of the following veggie combinations: broccoli and/or cauliflower florets; chopped green, red and/or yellow peppers; julienned zucchini, carrots and/or green onions. Sprinkle with a little marinade or white wine. Bake or microwave as directed. If microwaving, add an extra minute or two for the veggies.*

- ***Salsa Chicken in a Pouch:*** *Prepare Lemon Dill Chicken as directed, topping each chicken breast with 2 or 3 tablespoons homemade or bottled salsa. Wrap in parchment; bake or microwave as directed.*

Oven-Roasted Turkey Breast

An excellent alternative when you don't need a whole turkey.

1 turkey breast, bone in (about 3–3½ lb/1.5 kg)
salt, to taste
freshly ground pepper
3 cloves garlic, crushed
1 tbsp olive oil
1 tbsp Dijon mustard (optional)
2 tbsp balsamic vinegar or lemon juice
2 tbsp brown sugar or honey
1 tsp dried basil
1 tsp paprika
2 onions, sliced
½ cup water

1. Loosen skin from turkey, but don't remove it. Trim off fat. Season turkey breast under the skin with a little salt and pepper. In a small bowl, combine garlic with remaining ingredients except onions and water. Rub mixture over turkey breast (under the skin).
2. Place onions and water in the bottom of a lightly sprayed casserole. Place turkey, bone-side down, over onions. Cover and marinate for an hour at room temperature or 24 hours in the refrigerator.
3. Preheat oven to 350°F. Roast turkey uncovered for 50 to 60 minutes, basting every 20 minutes. Calculate 18–20 minutes per pound as your cooking time. After cooking, let turkey stand for 10 to 15 minutes for easier carving. Discard skin. Slice turkey meat on an angle off the bone.

Yield: 8 servings. Cooked turkey may become dry if frozen and reheated.

202 calories per serving, 2.7 g fat (0.5 g saturated), 97 mg cholesterol, 36 g protein, 7 g carbohydrate, 64 mg sodium, 410 mg potassium, 2 mg iron, <1 g fiber, 29 mg calcium.

Notes and Variations:

- *Fat-Saving Secrets! Cooking turkey with the skin on does not add more calories or fat. If desired, place thin slices of orange just under the skin to help keep turkey moist during cooking. Discard turkey skin and orange slices after cooking. Place casserole with cooking juices in the freezer for a short time so the fat will rise to the top and congeal, making it easy to remove.*
- ***Oven-Roasted Chicken Breasts:*** *Follow recipe for turkey breast, using 8 skinless, boneless chicken breasts. Reduce water to ¼ cup. Preheat oven to 400°F. Roast chicken uncovered for 20 to 25 minutes, basting occasionally. One serving contains 186 calories, 4.8 grams fat (1.1 grams saturated) and 73 milligrams cholesterol.*
- *The above seasoning mixture is also excellent for a rolled boneless turkey roast.*

Rozie's Freeze with Ease Turkey Chili

(See recipe, page 145.)

Sweet and Sour Stuffed Peppers

Sheila Denton suggested adding honey and lemon juice to the sauce. A grated apple can be added, too.

6 peppers (green and/or red)
1½ lb (750 g) lean ground turkey breast
2 egg whites (or 1 egg)
1 onion, minced
½ tsp salt
¼ tsp pepper
½ tsp dried basil
½ cup uncooked rice
2 cups tomato sauce

¼ cup honey
¼ cup lemon juice
1 bay leaf

1.   Cut tops off the peppers; carefully remove seeds and cores. Bring a large pot of water to a boil. Add peppers and simmer for 5 minutes, until softened. Drain well. Meanwhile, combine ground turkey with egg whites, onion, seasonings and rice.

2.   Combine tomato sauce, honey, lemon juice and bay leaf in a large pot; bring to a boil. Add ½ cup of sauce to the turkey mixture. Stuff the peppers and place them in a single layer in the pot. Reduce heat and simmer covered for 1½ to 2 hours, basting occasionally. Discard bay leaf.

Yield: 6 servings. These reheat and/or freeze well.

291 calories per serving, 1.2 g fat (0.3 g saturated), 70 mg cholesterol, 32 g protein, 38 g carbohydrate, 784 mg sodium, 838 mg potassium, 3 mg iron, 3 g fiber, 44 mg calcium.

■ BEEF

Cola Brisket

Brisket is quite high in fat, so serve it on special occasions. Cola makes the meat very tender.

3 onions, sliced
4½–5 lb beef brisket, well trimmed
4 cloves garlic, crushed
salt and pepper, to taste
1 tsp dried basil
1 tbsp paprika
¼ cup apricot jam
2 tbsp lemon juice
1 cup diet cola

1. Spray a large roasting pan with non-stick spray. Place onions in pan; place brisket on top of onions. Rub meat on all sides with garlic, seasonings, jam and lemon juice. Pour cola over and around brisket. Marinate for an hour at room temperature or overnight in the refrigerator.
2. Preheat oven to 325°F. Cook covered. Allow 45 minutes per pound as the cooking time, until meat is fork tender. Uncover meat for the last hour and baste it occasionally. Remove from oven and cool completely. Refrigerate overnight, if possible. Discard hardened fat that congeals on the surface. Slice brisket thinly across the grain, trimming away any fat. Reheat slices in the defatted pan juices.

Yield: 12 servings. Reheats and/or freezes well.

293 calories per serving, 14.3 g fat (6.4 g saturated), 103 mg cholesterol, 33 g protein, 6 g carbohydrate, 84 mg sodium, 385 mg potassium, 3 mg iron, <1 g fiber, 19 mg calcium.

Sweet and Sour BBQ Brisket

3 onions, sliced
4½–5 lb beef brisket, well trimmed
3 cloves garlic, crushed
1 tsp paprika
1 cup salsa
3 tbsp honey
2 tbsp lemon juice

1. Spray a large roasting pan with non-stick spray. Place onions in pan. Place brisket on top of onions and rub with garlic and paprika. Combine remaining ingredients and spread mixture over brisket. Marinate brisket for 1 hour at room temperature or overnight in the refrigerator.

2. Preheat oven to 325°F. Cook covered for 45 minutes per pound, until meat is fork tender. Uncover meat for the last hour and baste occasionally. Cool completely. Refrigerate overnight, if possible. Discard congealed fat. Slice brisket thinly across the grain, trimming away fat. Reheat slices in the defatted pan juices.

Yield: 12 servings. Reheats and/or freezes well.

300 calories per serving, 14.3 g fat (6.4 g saturated), 103 mg cholesterol, 33 g protein, 8 g carbohydrate, 137 mg sodium, 410 mg potassium, 3 mg iron, <1 g fiber, 24 mg calcium.

■ MARINADES AND SAUCES

Orange Balsamic Vinaigrette
Perfect for chicken. See recipe, page 106.

Roasted Red Pepper Coulis
Serve this vitamin-packed, fat-free sauce with fish, chicken, or vegetables.

   2–3 large roasted red peppers (homemade* or from a jar), chopped
   1 clove garlic, crushed
   1 medium onion, chopped
   1½ cups vegetable or chicken broth
   2–3 drops Tabasco sauce, optional
   salt and pepper, to taste
   1 tbsp fresh basil, minced (or ½ tsp dried)

1. In a medium saucepan, combine roasted peppers, garlic, onion and broth. Bring to a boil, reduce heat and simmer for 5 minutes. Cool slightly. Purée sauce. Add remaining ingredients and mix well. If sauce is too thick, add a little more broth or water. Serve warm.

Yield: About 1 cup sauce (4 servings). Sauce will keep for a day or two in the refrigerator.

27 calories per ¼ cup serving, 0.4 g fat (0 g saturated), 0 mg cholesterol, 1 g protein, 6 g carbohydrate, 252 sodium, 106 mg potassium, trace iron, <1 g fiber, 11 mg calcium.

*See recipe for Roasted Red Peppers (page 238). If using roasted peppers from a jar, you'll need about 1½ cups. However, they're higher in sodium.

Yogurt Dill Sauce

Delicious with fish, or use it as a creamy-style salad dressing.

> ½ cup fat-free or light mayonnaise
> ½ cup non-fat yogurt or sour cream
> 1 tbsp fresh lemon or lime juice
> 2 tbsp fresh dill, minced
> 2 tbsp green onion, minced
> salt and pepper, to taste

1. Combine mayonnaise, yogurt, lemon or lime juice, dill and green onion. Season to taste with salt and pepper. Chill before serving.

Yield: About 1 cup sauce.

8 calories per tbsp, 0 g fat (0 g saturated), trace cholesterol, trace protein, 2 g carbohydrate, 50 mg sodium, 22 mg potassium, 0 mg iron, 0 g fiber, 14 mg calcium.

■ PASTA

Also refer to Perfect Pasta-Bilities, chapter 5, page 146.

Best-O-Pesto
(See recipe, page 148.)

Cheater's Hi-Fiber Pasta Sauce
(See recipe, page 150.)

Cheater's Pasta
(See recipe, page 151.)

Fasta Pasta
(See recipe, page 151.)

Hi-Fiber Vegetarian Lasagna
(See recipe, page 152.)

Mexican Pasta with Beans
(See recipe, page 155.)

Penne Al Pesto Jardiniere
(See recipe, page 156.)

Penne with Roasted Peppers and Sun-Dried Tomatoes
(See recipe, page 158.)

Quick 'n Easy Tomato Sauce
(See recipe, page 159.)

Roasted Tomato, Garlic and Basil Sauce
(See recipe, page 161.)

Simple 'n Spicy Spirals
(See recipe, page 162.)

Spaghetti with Roasted Tomato, Garlic and Basil Sauce
(See recipe, page 162.)

Sun-Dried Tomato Pesto
(See recipe, page 163.)

Vegetarian Pad Thai
(See recipe, page 164.)

■ VEGETARIAN ENTREÉS

VEGETARIAN PLEASURES
- About 14 million North Americans consider themselves vegetarians. Of these, about one-third eliminate meat, fish and poultry from their diets. Some avoid red meat but include poultry or fish.
- There are many reasons for a vegetarian diet and lifestyle: health, environment, love of animals, concern for world hunger, belief in non-violence.
- A "real vegetarian" is someone who won't eat anything with either a face or a mother!
- Vegans don't eat any animal products, including meat, poultry, eggs and dairy products. Some won't eat honey. Many vegans won't use animal products such as leather or wool.
- Ovo-Lacto-Vegetarians eat both eggs and milk products. Lacto-Vegetarians

eat milk products but no eggs. Ovo-Vegetarians include eggs but exclude milk products from their diet.

- Part-time or "almost" vegetarians eat small amounts of animal protein (mainly chicken and/or fish once or twice a week) and lots of pasta; they also consume skim-milk dairy products and egg whites. (That's me!)

- The key to a healthy vegetarian diet is the same as any other healthy diet. Eat a wide variety of foods including fruits, vegetables, legumes, whole grains and small amounts of nuts and seeds.

- A plant-based diet is cholesterol free. It's also low in both total and saturated fats, except for nuts, seeds, oils and avocados.

- A mixture of proteins each day should provide enough essential amino acids. Most of us eat too much protein. You can get enough protein from plant foods by making healthful choices.

- Don't worry about eating enough protein. Each day, include some grains (barley, rice, kasha, couscous, pasta, bulgur, quinoa) and some legumes (lima, white or black beans, lentils, chickpeas, black-eyed peas, split peas). These don't have to be eaten at the same time. Just eat them on the same day, within a few hours of each other (e.g., Healthier Hummus on page 278, with a pita).

- Tofu (bean curd) and textured vegetable protein (TVP) are two other meat replacements. TVP is combined with water and used as a replacement for ground beef in recipes.

- Many people believe that starchy foods are fattening. Not true! Actually, carbohydrates are low in fat. It's the oil, butter, margarine or creamy sauces we add to them that are fattening. Portion distortion is also a big problem. If you eat too many calories, you'll end up with "thighs of regret!"

- "Lite" or low-fat margarine may contain gelatin, which is usually an animal-based product. Vegetarians and Kosher cooks should check labels carefully. Choose olive or canola oil instead of margarine whenever possible.

- Non-animal sources of iron include dried beans, lentils, leafy greens (spinach, Swiss chard, beet greens), bulgur, almonds, blackstrap molasses, prunes, apricots, raisins and other dried fruit.

- To increase the amount of iron absorbed at a meal, include foods with vitamin C (e.g., oranges or other citrus fruits, strawberries, melons, tomatoes, peppers, broccoli). It's best to eat foods that are high in iron and calcium at different times to increase iron absorption. Cooking food in cast iron cookware also adds to iron intake.
- Vitamin B12 is important for proper nervous system function. It comes primarily from animal-derived foods. A diet containing some egg or dairy products provides adequate vitamin B12.
- Fortified foods (e.g., cereals and pastas) are good non-animal sources of Vitamin B12. Check labels for products fortified with B12. You can also take a good multivitamin containing B12.

Belle's Chunky Ratatouille
(See recipe, page 165.)

Black Bean and Corn Casserole
(See recipe, page 166.)

Easy Enchiladas
(See recipe, page 168.)

Easy Vegetarian Chili
(See recipe, page 169.)

Enchilada Lasagna
(See recipe, page 172.)

Simple and Good Ratatouille (Mediterranean Vegetable Stew)
(See recipe, page 176.)

Vegetarian Cabbage Rolls
These taste great!

>Rainbow Rice Pilaf (see page 204)
>1 medium cabbage (about 3 lb/1.2 kg)
>boiling water
>19 oz can (540 ml) tomatoes
>5½ oz can (156 ml) tomato paste
>¼ cup brown sugar, packed
>2 tbsp lemon juice
>1 large onion, chopped

1. Prepare Rainbow Rice Pilaf as directed; let cool. Meanwhile, remove 12 of the large outer leaves from cabbage. Trim away tough ribs. Place cabbage leaves into a large pot of boiling water. Remove pot from heat, cover and let stand for 10 minutes. Drain cabbage thoroughly and set aside.
2. In the same pot, combine tomatoes, tomato paste, brown sugar and lemon juice. Break up tomatoes with a spoon. Remove ½ cup of sauce from pot and add it to rice mixture. Mix well.
3. Bring sauce mixture to a boil. Slice any leftover cabbage and add it to the sauce along with the chopped onion. Meanwhile, place a large spoonful of rice mixture on each cabbage leaf. Roll up, folding in ends. Carefully place cabbage rolls seam-side down in simmering sauce. Cook on low heat, partially covered, about 1 hour, until juice has thickened. Adjust seasonings to taste.

Yield: 12 cabbage rolls. These reheat well. Freezing is not recommended.

159 calories per cabbage roll, 1.7 g fat (0.2 g saturated), 0 mg cholesterol, 5 g protein, 34 g carbohydrate, 372 mg sodium, 479 mg potassium, 2 mg iron, 5 g fiber, 70 mg calcium.

Notes:

- *Crushed or diced canned tomatoes can be used. If you only have a very large can of tomatoes on hand, either freeze the leftovers or add them to your next vegetable soup or pasta sauce!*
- *Veggie Variations: If you have frozen tofu on hand, defrost and crumble it. You'll need about 1 cup. Combine crumbled tofu with rice mixture. Add salt, pepper and basil to taste. Stuff cabbage as directed. Another variation is to add 1 cup cooked or canned lentils or chickpeas.*
- *For other ideas for fillings, see notes following Vegetarian Stuffed Peppers.*

Vegetarian Stuffed Peppers

Easy, delicious and colorful.

> Rainbow Rice Pilaf (see page 204)
> 6 peppers (green, red, yellow and/or orange)
> 4 cups water
> 1½ cups tomato sauce (bottled or homemade)

1. Prepare Rainbow Rice Pilaf as directed, using vegetable broth. Cut peppers in half lengthwise through stem end. Carefully remove seeds and core. In a large saucepan, bring water to a boil. Add peppers and simmer for 3 or 4 minutes, until slightly softened. Drain well. Preheat oven to 350°F. Fill peppers with rice mixture. Spread 1 cup sauce on the bottom of a sprayed Pyrex oblong casserole. Arrange peppers in a single layer over sauce. Drizzle lightly with remaining sauce. Bake uncovered for 25 minutes (or microwave uncovered on HIGH for 12 to 15 minutes), until peppers are tender and heated through.

Yield: 6 servings as a main dish or 12 servings as a side dish. Reheats well. Do not freeze.

232 calories per main dish serving, 2.5 g fat (0.4 g saturated), 0 mg cholesterol, 7 g protein, 48 g carbohydrate, 727 mg sodium, 586 mg potassium, 3 mg iron, 5 g fiber, 52 mg calcium.

Variations:

- *Add ½ cup diced tofu to cooked rice for additional protein. For additional soluble fiber, add ½ cup canned red kidney beans or chickpeas, rinsed and drained. For additional calcium and protein, top each pepper with 2 tablespoons grated low-fat Swiss, Parmesan or mozzarella cheese during the last 10 minutes of baking (or the last 5 minutes of microwaving).*
- ***Stuffed Vegetables:*** *Any of the above fillings can be used to stuff Vegetarian Cabbage Rolls (page 244). Other veggies that are lovely when stuffed are hollowed-out tomatoes, zucchini or yellow squash halves. Use your imagination!*

DESSERTS

WHAT'S INSIDE

LOW GI SWEET DELIGHTS

- Life is short, so eat dessert first! There's still room in our lives for a little decadence. If you're faced with temptation, your best choice is a dessert based on fresh fruits. Limit rich desserts, but if you must indulge, eat a small portion, very, very slowly! Savor every mouthful.
- The average North American consumes 1½ pounds of sugar a week. How sweet life is! Sugar is a simple carbohydrate, which is hidden in many prepared foods. It has little in the way of nutrients.
- Decrease the sugar called for in your favorite recipes. Start with a 25 percent reduction, then taste to see if flavour and texture have been compromised. Sometimes sugar can be reduced by up to 50 percent.
- You can substitute liquid sugar substitute for liquid sugar (e.g., honey, maple syrup, molasses). But you cannot substitute granulated sugar with granulated substitutes, as they're usually higher GI than sugar. See Artificial Sweetener Rules (page 20).
- Fructose is a sweetener derived from the natural sugars in fruit, honey and invert sugar. It's 1½ times sweeter than sugar and is metabolized more slowly. Fructose is found in natural food stores.
- Fruit purées like unsweetened applesauce and Prune Purée (page 65) will lower the fat by at least half. As a bonus, Prune Purée is loaded with fiber!
- Health experts recommend 20 to 35 grams of fiber a day. Add oat bran, wheat bran and wheat germ to muffins, quickbreads, cookies and toppings for fruit crisps.
- To increase the fiber and tenderness of baked goods, replace half of the flour with whole-wheat flour. Another way to make baked goods more nutritious is to remove 2 tablespoons all-purpose flour from each cup called for in the recipe and replace with soy flour or wheat germ.
- Decrease the fat in your favorite recipes. Use non-fat or low-fat products wherever possible.
- Buttermilk, yogurt and low-fat sour cream can be substituted for each other in baking.

- Buttermilk is similar in fat content to skim milk, despite its high-fat name!
- Substitute skim or 1% milk (or evaporated skim milk) for whole milk for baking and desserts.
- Use non-stick vegetable spray to coat baking pans. However, sprays are made mainly from vegetable oils. A one-third second spray contains over a ¼ gram of fat, so spray lightly, my friend!
- Non-stick baking pans are great for low-fat baking and easy cleaning. If using dark or glass baking pans, lower the oven temperature called for in the recipe by 25°F.
- Read Baking the Low Fat and Low GI Way (page 261) and Substitutions and Alternatives in Low-Fat, Low-Cholesterol Baking (pages 264–266) for more ideas on low-fat baking techniques.
- Beware of high GI flour with unopposing soluble fibre. Using flour is fine when there are other ingredients that lower the GI content.
- Rolled oats can only have an opposing effect on the GI if it they are indeed rolled oats, not quick-cooking.
- Instead of using high GI cornstarch as a thickening agent, flour or oatbran can be used instead.
- Beware the use of high GI sweetening agents such as corn syrup, icing sugar or condensed milk without opposing soluble fibre to decrease the GI value of the recipe.
- All pastries with white flour only are considered high GI, even though the fat content is markedly improved compared to regular pastry.

RULES FOR ARTIFICIAL SWEETENERS IN LOW GI BAKING

Powdered sugar substitutes or sweeteners should not be used, as they contain high amounts of maltodextrin, a high GI bulking agent. Thus these sweeteners have a higher GI than sugar itself. However, liquid sweeteners usually do not contain maltodextrin, and neither do tablet sweeteners. Tablet sweeteners need only be dissolved in a very small quantity of water and added to the recipe. If bulk is required for the recipe, it's preferable to use sugar or fructose than powdered sugar substitutes or sweeteners.

■ CHOCOLATE

Chocolate and Mint Leaves

Unlike most other chocolate leaves, these are unique because the leaf is eaten together with the chocolate coating! Mint leaves are edible. Have a little folacin with your chocolate!

> 3 oz bittersweet or semisweet chocolate
> 18 large, fresh mint leaves

1. Melt chocolate on low heat in a double boiler. (Or microwave chocolate on MEDIUM power for 2 minutes; stir. Then microwave on MEDIUM 1 minute longer, until barely melted.) Let cool to just below body temperature, stirring occasionally.
2. Meanwhile, wash mint leaves thoroughly. Dry very well with paper towels. Line a cookie sheet with aluminum foil. Dip mint leaf completely in melted chocolate. Both sides of the leaf should be coated. Let excess chocolate drip back into the bowl. Place leaves on foil-lined tray and refrigerate until set. Use to decorate the top of cheesecake and around edges of serving plate.

Yield: 18 leaves. These will keep in the refrigerator up to 2 days.

20 calories per leaf, 1.7 g fat (0.9 g saturated), 0 mg cholesterol, trace protein, 2 g carbohydrate, trace sodium, 26 mg potassium, trace iron, trace fiber, 3 mg calcium.

Chocolate Chip Bran-ana Muffins

You won't taste the bran in these yummy muffins. What a great way to sneak in some extra fiber! Fruit, cereal and milk all come together in one healthy handful. Do try the variations listed.

> 1 cup All-Bran or natural bran cereal
> 1 cup buttermilk or sour milk

1 cup mashed ripe bananas (about 2 large)

2 egg whites (or 1 egg)

2 tbsp canola oil

2 tbsp unsweetened applesauce

½ cup sugar (brown or white)

1 cup all-purpose flour

½ cup whole-wheat flour

1 tsp baking powder

1 tsp baking soda

1 tsp cinnamon

¼–½ cup miniature chocolate chips

2 tbsp wheat germ, optional

1. Preheat oven to 375°F. Combine cereal with buttermilk in a large bowl. Let stand 3 or 4 minutes to soften. Add bananas, egg whites, oil and applesauce to bran mixture; blend well. Add remaining ingredients and stir just until blended. Do not over-mix. Spoon batter into paper-lined muffin cups, filling them ¾-full. Bake at 375°F for 20 to 25 minutes, until golden brown.

Yield: 12 muffins. These freeze very well.

174 calories per muffin, 3.9 g fat (1 g saturated), <1 mg cholesterol, 4 g protein, 34 g carbohydrate, 270 mg sodium, 280 mg potassium, 2 mg iron, 4 g fiber, 68 mg calcium.

Notes:

- *To make sour milk, mix 1 tablespoon lemon juice or vinegar with enough skim milk to equal 1 cup.*
- *You can replace the chocolate chips with ½ cup raisins or chopped dates. Chopped walnuts or almonds are another healthy option.*

Variations:

- **Fat-Free Bran-ana Muffins:** *Substitute ¼ cup Prune Purée (page 65) for oil and applesauce. Omit chocolate chips. (If desired, add ½ cup raisins or chopped dates.) Spray muffin pans with non-stick cooking spray. If you use paper liners, they should be sprayed before filling; otherwise muffins may stick because of the lack of fat in the batter.*
- **A-B-C Muffins (Applesauce, Apricot, Bran and Chocolate Chips):** *Substitute applesauce for mashed bananas. Add ½ cup chopped dried apricots to batter.*
- **A-B-C-D Muffins (Applesauce, Bran, Chocolate Chips and Dates):** *Substitute applesauce for mashed bananas. Add ½ cup chopped dates to batter.*
- **C-B-A Muffins (Cranberry, Bran and Applesauce):** *Substitute applesauce for mashed bananas. Soak ½ cup of dried cranberries in hot water for 5 to 10 minutes, then drain well before adding them to the batter. (To use fresh or frozen cranberries, mix 1 cup of berries with 1 tablespoon flour and 2 tablespoons sugar. Gently mix into batter.)*
- **Mini-Muffins:** *Prepare desired batter (above). Pour into paper lined mini-muffin tins. Bake at 375°F for 15 to 18 minutes. Recipe makes 3 dozen minis. Three minis equal 1 regular muffin.*

Hot Chocolate (Cocoa)

Whenever I have a craving for chocolate or need to lower my stress level, I have a cup of cocoa and it feels like a warm hug! It also helps you sleep better if you have a cup before bedtime. Calci-yummy!

    1 tsp unsweetened cocoa
    1 cup skim milk
    sugar or low GI sweetener to taste (quantity varies on the manufacturer)

1.   Measure cocoa in a microsafe mug. Add a little milk and stir to make a smooth paste. Gradually stir in remaining milk. Microwave on HIGH for 2 minutes, until steaming hot, stirring once or twice. Stir in sugar Makes 1 cup.

122 calories per serving (with sugar), 0.7 g fat (0.4 g saturated), 4 mg cholesterol, 9 g protein, 21 g carbohydrate, 127 mg sodium, 434 mg potassium, trace iron, <1 g fiber, 304 mg calcium.

■ CHILLED OR FROZEN DISHES

Chunky Monkey

Packed with potassium and fiber, plus 232 mg of calcium, what a yummy breakfast or snack!

¾ cup skim milk
½ of a frozen banana
1 tsp cocoa
2–3 ice cubes
sugar or low GI sweetener to taste (quantity depends on brand)

1.   In a blender or processor, blend the first 4 ingredients together until smooth. Add sweetener to taste. Makes 1 serving.

155 calories per serving (with sugar), 0.9 g fat (0.5 g saturated), 3 mg cholesterol, 7 g protein, 32 g carbohydrate, 96 mg sodium, 566 mg potassium, <1 mg iron, 2 g fiber, 232 mg calcium.

Fruit Smoothies

(See recipe, page 51.)

Mock Banana Soft Ice Cream

2 large ripe bananas, sliced
½ cup non-fat cottage cheese or part-skim ricotta cheese
½ tsp vanilla
4 tsp sugar

1. Arrange banana slices in a single layer on a waxed-paper lined plate. Cover and freeze until firm. Frozen slices can be frozen in a tightly sealed container for up to a month. (I've also frozen whole bananas in their skins, then removed them from the freezer at serving time and placed them under running water for 30 seconds. Peel with a sharp knife and cut into chunks.) At serving time, combine ingredients in the processor and process until smooth. Serve immediately.

Yield: 4 servings.

102 calories per serving, 0.3 g fat (0.1 g saturated), 3 mg cholesterol, 5 g protein, 22 g carbohydrate, 93 mg sodium, 300 mg potassium, trace iron, 2 g fiber, 19 mg calcium.

Variations:

- ***Mock Banana-Strawberry Soft Ice Cream:*** *Follow the recipe above, using 1 banana and 1½ cups ripe strawberries. One serving contains 82 calories and 16 grams carbohydrate.*
- ***Easiest Frozen Banana Mousse:*** *Peel and slice 4 ripe bananas. Arrange in a single layer on a plate and cover tightly to prevent them from absorbing any odors. Freeze completely. When needed, thaw for 5 minutes, then process with 1 teaspoon of lemon juice in the processor until smooth. Serve immediately. Makes 4 servings.*

Orange Creamy Dream

Packed with potassium!

½ cup frozen concentrated orange juice
2½ cups skim milk
1 cup non-fat yogurt
1 tsp vanilla extract
2–3 ice cubes
low GI sweetener to taste (quantity depends on brand)

1. Blend all ingredients together until smooth. Makes 5 servings.

119 calories per serving, 0.4 g fat (0.2 g saturated), 3 mg cholesterol, 8 g protein, 21 g carbohydrate, 102 mg sodium, 521 mg potassium, trace iron, 2 g fiber, 257 mg calcium.

Strawberry and Banana Frozen Yogurt

(See recipe, page 56.)

Strawberry Buttermilk Sherbet

So pretty, so delicious! Leftover buttermilk can be used in muffin or cake recipes.

1½–2 cups frozen strawberries
¼ cup sugar or honey
¼–⅓ cup buttermilk
1 tsp lemon juice

1. Process berries with sugar until you get the texture of snow. Gradually add buttermilk and lemon juice through the feed tube. Process until well mixed and the texture of sherbet. Serve immediately.

Yield: 3 to 4 servings. Recipe can be doubled easily.

99 calories per serving, 0.3 g fat (0.1 g saturated), <1 mg cholesterol, 1 g protein, 25 g carbohydrate, 23 mg sodium, 144 mg potassium, <1 mg iron, 2 g fiber, 36 mg calcium.

Notes:
- *Either use 1 package of frozen unsweetened strawberries (about 1½ cups), or freeze 2 cups of very ripe strawberries for this recipe. The more berries you use, the more buttermilk you need to add.*
- *Raspberries can be used instead of strawberries. No-fat yogurt can be used instead of buttermilk.*

Strawberry Surprise

One cup of strawberries contains 85 milligrams of vitamin C—more than an orange! Strawberries are packed with antioxidants and contain virtually no fat. One cup of berries contains 46 calories and more than 3 grams of fiber. Now that's very berry good news, and so are the desserts that follow!

3 cups non-fat natural yogurt (without gelatin or stabilizers)
4 cups ripe strawberries, hulled and sliced
2–3 tbsp orange liqueur (e.g., Sabra)
3 tbsp maple syrup or honey (to taste)

1. Line a strainer with a paper coffee filter, paper towelling or a cheesecloth. Place strainer over a large glass measuring cup or bowl. Spoon yogurt into strainer and let drain for 1 hour, or until yogurt has reduced to 2 cups. (Drained whey can be used instead of buttermilk or yogurt in baking.)
2. Sprinkle strawberries with liqueur and marinate for 30 minutes; drain. Fold half of berries into thickened yogurt. Sweeten to taste. Layer remaining berries and yogurt mixture in 6 parfait or wine glasses, starting and ending with berries. Chill before serving.

Yield: 6 servings. Leftovers can be refrigerated for up to 2 days if well covered.

131 calories per serving, 0.6 g fat (0.1 g saturated), 2 mg cholesterol, 7 g protein, 24 g carbohydrate, 60 mg sodium, 382 mg potassium, trace iron, 2 g fiber, 171 mg calcium.

Variations:

- *If you don't have any orange liqueur on hand, substitute 2 tablespoons of white wine and 1 tablespoon orange juice. If desired, arrange a layer of peeled, sliced kiwis as the middle layer.*
- **Strawberry Pudding Parfaits:** *Instead of yogurt, substitute 1 package (6 serving size) vanilla pudding mix. Cook according to package directions, using skim milk. Stir 1 tablespoon of orange liqueur into cooked pudding. Cover to prevent a skin from forming; chill. Layer marinated strawberries and pudding in parfait glasses. Chill before serving.*
- **Strawberry and Ice Cream Parfaits:** *Instead of drained yogurt, substitute low-fat ice cream (strawberry or vanilla) or frozen yogurt. Layer marinated strawberries and ice cream in parfait glasses. Serve immediately. (This is also scrumptious if you prepare the yogurt/berry mixture as directed in the main recipe and use it as a topping over the ice cream and strawberries!)*

■ FRUIT DESSERTS

Barbecue Fruit 'n Cream

Easy and decadent. Calci-yummy!

> 3 tbsp maple syrup
> 2 cups sliced fresh peaches, nectarines and/or pears
> 2 cups vanilla frozen low-fat yogurt

1. Drizzle maple syrup over fruit. Wrap in heavy-duty aluminum foil, seal well to make a package and heat for 20 minutes on the dying embers of your BBQ. Serve piping hot over frozen yogurt.

Yield: 4 servings. Leftover fruit can be refrigerated for a day or two and reheated in the microwave.

236 calories per serving, 2.6 g fat (1.5 g saturated), 45 mg cholesterol, 9 g protein, 46 g carbohydrate, 56 mg sodium, 198 mg potassium, trace iron, 2 g fiber, 308 mg calcium.

Citrus or Melon Baskets

(See recipe, page 50.)

Homemade Applesauce

(See recipe, page 52.)

Jumbleberry Crisp

(See recipe, page 53.)

Melons and Berries in Wine

A light and refreshing dessert, loaded with potassium and fiber.

> 1½ cups medium white wine
> 2 tbsp honey or sugar
> 2–3 slices ginger root
> ½ of a medium cantaloupe, halved and seeded
> ½ of a honeydew, seeded
> ½ of a Casaba or Crenshaw melon, seeded
> 2 cups fresh strawberries, hulled and halved
> 1–2 cups fresh blueberries

1. In a saucepan, combine wine with honey and ginger. Bring to a boil, reduce heat and simmer uncovered for 5 minutes. Remove from heat and let cool to room temperature. Discard ginger.
2. Use a melon baller to scoop out balls from the melons. Place in a large bowl along with the strawberries and blueberries. Pour the cooled wine over fruit and mix gently. Refrigerate for 1 to 2 hours to blend the flavors. Spoon fruit into chilled serving dishes. Drizzle wine over fruit.

Yield: 8 servings.

162 calories per serving, 0.6 g fat (0.1 g saturated), 0 mg cholesterol, 3 g protein, 33 g carbohydrate, 40 mg sodium, 876 mg potassium, 1 mg iron, 4 g fiber, 30 mg calcium.

Note:

- *Half a cantaloupe supplies nearly double the daily recommended intake of vitamin C. It will provide as much vitamin C as 1½ oranges. Cantaloupe is also a great source of beta carotene. So save the other half of the cantaloupe for a mega-healthy breakfast. The vitamin C in the melon enhances iron absorption from your bowl of cereal.*

Variations:

- ***Super Smoothie:*** *Combine the flesh of ½ cantaloupe, ½ melon, 1 banana, 8 strawberries and a few ice cubes in the blender or processor. Makes 2 servings.*

Peachy Crumb Crisp

(See recipe, page 55, and its variations for Blueberry Peach Crisp, Blueberry Nectarine Crisp, Apple Crisp, and Strawberry Rhubarb Crisp.)

Strawberries with Balsamic Vinegar or Red Wine

The natural sugars in the berries and vinegar make a yummy syrup. Always rinse berries before you remove the stems. Otherwise, berries will become waterlogged.

> 2 pints strawberries
> 1 tbsp orange juice or Grand Marnier
> 3 tbsp balsamic vinegar or red wine
> 3 tbsp brown sugar (or to taste)

1. Rinse, hull and slice berries. Mix gently with remaining ingredients. Refrigerate covered for at least a ½ hour. (The longer they stand, the more delicious they become.)

Yield: 4 to 6 servings.

94 calories per serving, 0.6 g fat (0 g saturated), 0 mg cholesterol, 1 g protein, 23 g carbohydrate, 8 mg sodium, 283 mg potassium, <1 mg iron, 3 g fiber, 31 mg calcium.

■ MUFFINS

Also refer to Muffinformation, pages 68–70, and Going Bananas, pages 74–76.

Apple Streusel Oatmeal Muffins
(See recipe, page 66.)

Bran and Date Muffins
(See recipe, page 66.)

Bran and Honey Muffins
(See recipe, page 70.)

Carolyn's Thin Muffin Loaf
(See recipe, page 72.)

Carrot Muffins
(See recipe, page 73.)

Mary's Best Bran-ana Bread
(See recipe, page 73.)

Rozie's Magical Carrot Muffins
(See recipe, page 75.)

Wheat Germ Bran Muffins
(See recipe, page 76.)

■ BAKING TIPS AND CAKES

BAKING THE LOW FAT AND LOW GI WAY

- For baking, because of health concerns, I've made the switch from butter to canola oil or tub margarine. I use either Fleishmann's tub margarine, which is dairy-free (pareve), or Becel tub margarine, which contains dairy. When I want the flavor of butter, I do indulge occasionally and use butter, but in very small amounts.
- Margarine is not less fattening than butter! It's just lower in saturated fats and cholesterol. Margarine and butter contain the same number of calories, about 100 per tablespoon.
- Reduced fat/low-calorie brands of margarine and butter are fine as spreads, but don't use them for baking. They contain 50 percent water, so they won't work properly in most baking recipes. However, I have used "lite" margarine in fruit crisp toppings with excellent results.
- In your traditional favorite baking recipes, you can reduce the fat by at least half by using fruit purées such as unsweetened applesauce or prunes (see Say "Hooray" for Prune Purée! below)
- Cakes made with butter or margarine get some of their volume from the air that's incorporated into the batter when you cream fat with sugar. If you eliminate all the fat from the recipe, your baked goods will be more compact. Start by replacing only half the fat in your recipe. Check out the results and if satisfactory, next time reduce the fat a little more.
- How low can you go? Use ⅓ of the amount of fat called for in the original recipe, and replace the remainder with fruit purée (e.g., instead of 1 cup oil, use ⅓ cup oil and ⅔ cup unsweetened applesauce or Prune Purée).
- When should you add the fat substitute? In most recipes, beat it together with the oil or margarine, sugar and flavoring. Baked goods may be slightly more dense than those made with the full amount of fat, but flavor and moistness are fine.

- To retain moistness when baking fat-free and fat-reduced items, I often reduce the oven temperature by 25 degrees to prevent over-baking. Test with a wooden skewer or toothpick. It should come out clean when inserted into the center.
- Quick Fixes: Dust cakes with a combination of cocoa and icing sugar. Place a doily, stencil or small cookie cutters on top of cake before sprinkling it with cocoa/sugar mixture.
- Sugar-free pudding (any flavor) makes a delicious icing for cakes!

SAY "HOORAY" FOR PRUNE PURÉE!

- Mention the word "prunes" and the usual associations that come to mind are prune juice, stewed prunes, hamentashen—and digestive systems in need of a little boost for regularity! Whenever I see prunes, I'm reminded of a song my sister and I used to sing as children: "No matter how young a prune may be, he's always full of wrinkles. A baby prune's just like his dad, but he's not wrinkled quite so bad! We have wrinkles on our face, a prune has wrinkles every place!"
- Well, that wrinkled old prune has become a boon to low-fat bakers. Invest just 5 minutes of your time and whip up an excellent fat replacement to use in most of your baking recipes. Prune Purée is high in pectin, a soluble fiber, which helps hold in the air bubbles, and also helps keep baked goods moist. It works well in your favorite chocolate cake, brownies, banana bread, carrot or zucchini muffins. Go ahead and experiment! Baked goods will have a slightly fruity taste, but no one will be able to guess that you've substituted prunes for fat.
- Add a little fiber to your diet by adding Prune Purée to home-baked goodies. One cup contains 12 grams of fiber! (What better excuse do you need to indulge in a brownie or two?)
- For light-colored cakes, Prune Purée can be combined with unsweetened applesauce.
- For best results, be sure to use some fat in your low-fat baking recipes.

Don't be tempted to replace all of the fat with fruit purée. Otherwise, the tops of baked goods usually end up being somewhat sticky and the texture can be a bit rubbery.

- A fat-free product called "Lighter Bake" is an excellent fat replacement for butter, margarine, oil and shortening. It can be used in moist, soft and chewy baking recipes or mixes. It's made from prunes, apples and pectin, and is used as a fat replacement in the same way you use prune purée or applesauce. It's manufactured by Sunsweet, 501 N. Walton Avenue, Yuba City, CA 95993. Call 800-417-2253 between 9 a.m. and 6 p.m. (PST) for information or recipes. From Canada, call their Consumer Relations department at 209-467-6260.

- Homemade Prune Purée (page 65) makes a delicious filling for many baked goods. If desired, add a teaspoon of grated orange or lemon rind (zest). It also makes a delicious fat-free spread on bread or toast instead of jam. So the plump little plum, even when it reaches old age, has found a new purpose in life. After all, what's a wrinkle or two between friends?

- Dare to Compare! One cup of Prune Purée contains 304 calories and less than 1 gram of fat. One cup of butter contains 1,628 calories and 184 grams of fat. One cup of oil contains 1,927 calories and 218 grams of fat!

SUBSTITUTIONS AND ALTERNATIVES IN LOW-FAT, LOW-CHOLESTEROL BAKING

FOR	USE
1 tbsp Butter	1 tbsp tub margarine, canola or walnut oil. (Light margarine can be used for streusel toppings, but not regular baking. Some light brands contain gelatin, an animal-based product, and may not be Kosher.)
1/2 cup butter, oil or margarine	3 tbsp canola oil or tub margarine plus ⅓ cup unsweetened applesauce, Prune Purée (page 65) or fruit purée fat replacer (e.g., Lighter Bake, sold in the U.S.)
1 cup butter, oil or margarine	⅓ cup canola oil or tub margarine plus ⅔ cup unsweetened applesauce or fruit purée fat replacer.
1 cup whole or 2% milk	1 cup skim milk or lactose-reduced milk/lactaid. (For dairy-free baking, use orange or apple juice, water, coffee, soymilk or rice milk.)
1 cup buttermilk or yogurt	1 tbsp lemon juice or vinegar plus skim milk to equal 1 cup.
1 cup sour cream	1 cup non-fat or low-fat sour cream or yogurt (or buttermilk).
1 cup cream cheese	1 cup dry cottage cheese (pressed or smooth texture) or ricotta cheese (non-fat/low-fat), Homemade Cottage Cheese (page 46) or low-fat cream cheese.

FOR	USE
2 cups whipped cream	Combine ⅓ cup ice water, 2 tsp lemon juice and ½ tsp vanilla in a deep bowl. Blend in ⅓ cup skim milk powder plus 2 tbsp sugar. Whip 5 to 10 minutes, until stiff.
1 cup sugar	Do not substitute with any powdered sweeteners as they usually contain Maltodextrin as a bulking agent. Maltodextrin is very high GI and to be avoided in all areas. See Rules for Artificial Sweeteners, page 20.
1 cup brown sugar, packed	1 cup granulated sugar plus 2 tbsp molasses.
1 cup all-purpose or unbleached flour	2 tbsp wheat germ or soy flour plus all-purpose flour to equal 1 cup. Or 1 cup sifted whole-wheat (or white) cake and pastry flour.
1 square unsweetened chocolate	3 tbsp unsweetened cocoa plus ½ tbsp canola oil.
1 egg (in baking or cooking)	2 egg whites or ¼ cup egg whites or egg substitute (or use omega-3-reduced-cholesterol eggs).
1 egg (in baking) (Vegan alternative)	¼ cup mashed banana, tofu or low-fat sour cream. Baked goods may be more dense and heavy than those with eggs.

FOR	USE
1 egg (in baking) (Vegan alternative)	Grind flax seed in a coffee grinder or spice mill (or buy flax seed already ground). For 1 egg, combine 1 tbsp ground flax seed with 3 tbsp water in a small bowl. Let stand until thick, about 2 or 3 minutes. Store flax seed in the freezer to avoid rancidity. Flax seed is high in essential omega-3 fatty acids.
Juice of a lemon	3 to 4 tbsp lemon juice (fresh or bottled).
Juice of an orange	¼ to ⅓ cup orange juice.
Juice of a lime	2 tbsp lime juice.
1 tsp baking powder	½ tsp cream of tartar plus ¼ tsp baking soda.
1/2 cup nuts	¼ cup finely chopped nuts. (Toast nuts at 350°F for 5 to 10 minutes before chopping to enhance flavor.) Supplement with 1/4 cup crunchy cereal (e.g., Grape Nuts).
1/2 cup raisins	½ cup dried cherries, blueberries, cranberries, strawberries, chopped dates, apricots, prunes (for muffins/baked goods).

Apple Streusel Oatmeal Cake
(See recipe, page 77.)

Mini Cheesecakes

These mini cheesecakes are so versatile. They're smooth and decadent tasting, yet low in fat. I like to make them with Yogurt Cheese (see below), which is fat-free and provides a wonderful creamy texture. Although cornstarch in most recipes is a high GI thickening agent, together with so much protein and a small amount of cornstarch, the GI is kept relatively low.

¼ cup non-fat sour cream (or 1½ cups non-fat yogurt)
1 lb (500 g) dry cottage cheese (non-fat)
¾ cup granulated sugar
2 eggs (or 1 egg plus 2 egg whites)
1 tbsp lemon juice
2 tsp cornstarch
½ cup reduced-sugar jam (or 1 cup fresh berries)

1. If using yogurt, place it in a strainer lined with a paper coffee filter. Place over a bowl and let drain for 3 to 4 hours. You will have ¼ cup of Yogurt Cheese.
2. Preheat oven to 350°F. Beat cottage cheese with sugar until smooth and creamy, about 1 to 2 minutes. Add sour cream or Yogurt Cheese, eggs, lemon juice and cornstarch. Mix just until blended.
3. Line 12 muffin tins with paper baking cups. Fill ¾-full with cheese mixture. Place muffin pan into a larger pan. Pour hot water into the larger pan to come halfway up the sides of the muffin pan. Bake at 350°F for 30 minutes, just until set. Cool to room temperature. Cover and chill for several hours or overnight. Top each cheesecake with a spoonful of your favorite jam. You could also use fresh blueberries, sliced strawberries or raspberries.

Yield: 12 mini cheesecakes. Do not freeze. These will keep for 2 or 3 days in the refrigerator.

117 calories per serving (with 2 tsp jam), 1 g fat (0.3 g saturated), 38 mg cholesterol, 6 g protein, 21 g carbohydrate, 132 mg sodium, 54 mg potassium, trace iron, trace fiber, 30 mg calcium.

Variations:
- ***Praline Cheesecakes:*** *Use firmly packed brown sugar instead of granulated sugar. Use 1 teaspoon vanilla instead of lemon juice. When cool, garnish each one with a pecan half.*

Moist 'n Luscious Carrot Cake
(See recipe, page 79.)

SNACKS

WHAT'S INSIDE

■ SNACKS YOU CAN BUY IN A CAN OR PACKAGE

There are many low GI snacks you can buy in a package. Here are some suggestions:

- Canned Fruits (not packed in syrup).
- Low fat cheeses (especially mini-cheeses).
- Dried fruits or vegetables, especially sun-dried tomatoes.
- Nuts, especially walnuts and nut bars, and natural peanut butter (with no added sugars).
- Marinated vegetables packed in jars. These are great as snacks and side dishes. An added benefit is the vinegar they contain, which helps lower the GI of the foods you eat along with them. Best picks: artichoke hearts, olives, capers, any marinated vegetable medley or mix, roasted peppers and any type of pickles.

RAW GI SNACKS

The lowest GI fruits to choose from include all varieties of citrus fruits (e.g., grapefruit, orange) as well as apples, apricots, cherries, mulberries, peaches, pears, plums, strawberries and kiwi fruit. Yellowish green bananas are fine, but riper bananas with brown spots are higher GI.

As for vegetables, most leafy green vegetables and cruciferous vegetables are low GI, including beans, lentils and chickpeas. Raw vegetables are perfect with dips and spreads listed in this chapter. See also Appendix A at the back of this book.

■ HOMEMADE CARBS

These are perfect for dips or spreads.

Belle's Flatbread (Lavasch)

This flatbread is a great alternative to packaged crackers. Luscious with soups, salads, dips and spreads.

1 cup flour
½ cup rolled oats
¼ tsp salt
1 tbsp onion flakes
2 tbsp sesame seeds
¼ tsp garlic powder
2 tbsp canola oil
6 tbsp water

1. Preheat oven to 475°F. Line 2 baking sheets with aluminum foil and spray with non-stick spray. Combine flour, rolled oats, seasonings and oil in the processor. Process until mixed. Slowly add water through the feed tube and process until mixture gathers together into a crumbly mass. Remove dough from processor and press it together to form a ball. Divide into 18 smaller balls.
2. On a floured surface, roll out each piece of dough as thin as possible into long strips. During the rolling process, sprinkle dough with desired toppings, pressing the toppings into the dough with the rolling pin. (Alternately, use a pasta machine to roll out dough.) Bake at 475°F for 5 to 6 minutes, until crisp and golden.

Optional Toppings: sesame seeds, coarse salt, dill weed, dried basil and/or dehydrated onion flakes.

Yield: 18 pieces. Store in an airtight container.

54 calories per piece, 2.2 g fat (0.1 g saturated), 0 mg cholesterol, 1 g protein, 7 g carbohydrate, 35 mg sodium, 19 mg potassium, <1 mg iron, <1 g fiber, 6 mg calcium.

Pita or Tortilla Chips

These are addictive! I used to brush them with oil, but was "de-lited" to find out that egg white worked perfectly! If making tortilla chips, try to buy tortillas with no added fat.

6 medium-size pitas or 12 thin tortillas (whole wheat or flour)
1–2 egg whites
salt, to taste
1–2 cloves garlic, crushed
dash of basil, oregano and/or thyme

1. Preheat oven to 400°F. If using pitas, split each into 2 rounds. Use a pastry brush to paint a light coating of egg white on one side. Sprinkle lightly with seasonings. Pile in a stack and use a sharp knife or pizza wheel to cut the stack into wedges. Arrange in a single layer on non-stick or sprayed baking sheet(s).
2. Bake at 400°F for 8 to 10 minutes, until crisp and golden. (Watch carefully to prevent burning.) Serve warm or at room temperature.

Yield: 12 servings. (Allow half a pita or 1 tortilla per serving.) These freeze well.

77 calories per serving, 0.5 g fat (0 g saturated), 0 mg cholesterol, 2 g protein, 15 g carbohydrate, 150 mg sodium, 5 mg potassium, <1 mg iron, 1 g fiber, 21 mg calcium.

Variations:
- ***Pita or Tortilla Ribbons:*** *Follow directions above, but cut pitas or tortillas into long narrow strips instead of wedges. (You can also sprinkle them with*

grated Parmesan cheese. For a spicy version, omit salt and spices; sprinkle with Cajun seasoning.)
- ***Make and Break Chips:*** *Follow directions above, but don't cut pitas or tortillas before baking. Bake at 400°F for 8 to 10 minutes. Break roughly into large pieces.*

Sweet Potato Chips

Packaged chips are full of fat, calories and sodium. One package supposedly contains 7 servings. Certainly not for any 7 people that I know! These crunchy munchies are easy and guilt-free.

> 1– 4 medium sweet potatoes, peeled, thinly sliced
> salt, to taste
> basil, oregano, garlic powder and/or cayenne, if desired

1. Scrub potatoes thoroughly; dry well. Slice paper thin, either in the processor or by hand. You should get about 24 slices from each potato. Cook in the microwave or conventional oven (below).

- *Microwave Method:* Place 12 slices at a time on a microsafe rack. Sprinkle lightly with desired seasonings. Microwave on HIGH for 4 minutes, or until dry and crunchy. Watch carefully because cooking time depends on moisture content of potatoes. If necessary, microwave 30 seconds longer and check again. Repeat until crispy. Repeat with remaining potato slices.
- *Conventional Method (for a large batch):* Preheat oven to 450°F. Spray a baking sheet lightly with non-stick spray. Place potato slices in a single layer on pan. Sprinkle lightly with seasonings. Bake at 450°F about 15 to 20 minutes, until crispy and golden.

Yield: Calculate ½ potato (about 12 chips) as 1 serving. Do not freeze.

59 calories per serving, 0.1 g fat (0 g saturated), 0 mg cholesterol, 1 g protein, 14 g carbohydrate, 6 mg sodium, 198 mg potassium, trace iron, 2 g fiber, 16 mg calcium.

Note:

- *These are best eaten within a few days. The fresher, the better! (They never last very long at my house!)*

Whole-Wheat Pitas

For hors d'oeuvres, make miniature pitas. Baking time will be 5 to 6 minutes.

    1 tsp sugar
    ¼ cup warm water (about 110°F)
    1 pkg active dry yeast
    1½ cups all-purpose flour
    1½ cups whole-wheat flour (approximately)
    1 tsp salt
    2 tsp additional sugar
    1 cup lukewarm water
    1 tsp canola oil

1. Dissolve sugar in warm water. Sprinkle yeast over water and let stand for 8 to 10 minutes, until foamy. Stir to dissolve. Combine flours, salt, additional sugar and yeast mixture in processor. Process for 8 to 10 seconds. Pour lukewarm water and oil through feed tube while machine is running. Process until dough is well kneaded and gathers in a mass around the blades, about 1 minute. If machine begins to slow down, add 2 or 3 tablespoons additional whole-wheat flour.

2. Transfer dough to a lightly floured surface. Knead dough for 2 minutes by hand, until smooth. Divide dough into 16 balls. Roll each ball into a circle about ¼ inch thick. Cover with a towel and let rise for a half hour. Roll out thinly once again and let rise a half-hour longer.

3. Preheat oven to 500°F. Place pitas on a lightly greased or sprayed baking sheet. Bake about 6 to 8 minutes, or until puffed up and golden. Insides of pita will be hollow. Cool on a rack. To fill, make a slit along one edge of pita and stuff as desired.

Yield: 16 pitas. These freeze very well.

88 calories per pita, 0.6 g fat (0.1 g saturated), 0 mg cholesterol, 3 g protein, 18 g carbohydrate, 147 mg sodium, 67 mg potassium, 1 mg iron, 2 g fiber, 6 mg calcium.

■ DIPS AND SPREADS

Use veggies or homemade carbs above with the following dips or spreads.

Babaganouj (Mediterranean Eggplant)
Tasty and colorful! The eggplant is broiled in this recipe, but it can be microwaved (see below).

> 1 large eggplant (about 1½ lb/750 g)
> 1 clove garlic, crushed
> 1 small tomato, chopped
> ½ of a green pepper, chopped
> 2–3 tbsp tahini (sesame paste)
> 3 tbsp fresh lemon juice
> salt and pepper, to taste
> ¼ tsp cumin, or to taste
> 2 tbsp non-fat yogurt, optional
> 2 tbsp chopped fresh parsley, to garnish

1. Preheat broiler. Cut eggplant in half. Pierce skin in several places with a fork. Place cut-side down on a broiler rack. Broil 4 inches from the heat for about 20 minutes. Do not turn eggplant over during cooking. Remove from oven and let cool. Squeeze gently to press out excess moisture. Scoop out pulp and mash well. Mix together with remaining ingredients except parsley. Place in a serving bowl; garnish with parsley. Served chilled with pita and/or crudités. Keeps 3 or 4 days in the fridge.

Yield: About 3 cups. If freezing, add tahini and yogurt after defrosting eggplant.

7 calories per tbsp, 0.3 g fat (0.1 g saturated), 0 mg cholesterol, trace protein, 1 g carbohydrate, <1 mg sodium, 37 mg potassium, trace iron, trace fiber, 2 mg calcium.

Note:

- *How to Microwave Eggplant: Wash eggplant and dry well. Pierce skin in several places with a fork. An average eggplant weighs about 1½ pounds and takes 7 to 8 minutes to cook. Place on a microsafe rack. Microwave uncovered on HIGH, allowing 5 to 6 minutes per pound. Halfway through cooking, turn eggplant over. At the end of cooking, it will be tender when pierced with a fork and will collapse slightly. Remove from microwave and let stand for 10 minutes. Cut in half and scoop out pulp. Sprinkle with a little lemon juice to keep the color light.*

Basic Skinny Dip

Use fresh dill for a simply dill-icious dip! Your processor will help you prepare this in a flash.

½ cup smooth non-fat cottage cheese
½ cup non-fat yogurt
¼ cup green onions, minced
¼ cup minced green pepper
2 tbsp grated carrots, optional
2 tbsp fresh dill, minced (or ½ tsp dried)
1 tsp lemon or lime juice
salt and pepper, to taste

1. Combine all ingredients and mix well. Chill until serving time. Serve with assorted vegetables.

Yield: About 1¼ cups. Keeps about 3 or 4 days in the refrigerator.

8 calories per tbsp, 0 g fat (0 g saturated), <1 g cholesterol, 1 g protein, <1 g carbo-hydrate, 22 mg sodium, 25 mg potassium, 0 mg iron, trace fiber, 15 mg calcium.

Note:

- *If using creamed cottage cheese, drain off excess liquid. Process cottage cheese until completely smooth, about 2 to 3 minutes in the processor. Add remaining ingredients. Blend in with quick on/offs.*

Variations:

- *Use basil instead of dill. Add 1 clove minced garlic, if desired. Substitute ¼ cup minced red pepper instead of green pepper. Use minced red onion instead of green onions.*

Creamy Salmon Paté (Mock Salmon Mousse)

(For recipe, see page 121)

Green Pea Guacamole

With this recipe, you won't have to worry about finding ripe avocados. Frozen green peas will be ready when you are, and they won't turn brown when mashed. One cup of green peas contains 111 calories and only half a gram of fat!

    1 cup frozen green peas
    1 clove garlic
    2–3 tsp fresh lime juice (to taste)
    3 tbsp mild or medium salsa
    3 tbsp non-fat yogurt or sour cream
    ½ tsp extra-virgin olive oil, optional
    salt and pepper, optional
    pinch of cumin

1. Microwave peas on HIGH for 2 minutes, just until defrosted. In the food processor, drop garlic through the feed tube and process until minced. Add lime juice and peas. Process until minced, about 1 minute, scraping down sides of bowl several times. Blend in salsa, yogurt and oil, if using. Season to taste. Transfer mixture to a bowl, cover and refrigerate until ready to serve. (Can be made up to 1 day in advance.)

Yield: About 1 cup. Do not freeze. Delicious as a dip with Pita or Tortilla Chips (see page 272).

9 calories per tbsp, 0 g fat (0 g saturated), 0 mg cholesterol, <1 g protein, 2 g carbohydrate, 19 mg sodium, 27 mg potassium, trace iron, <1 g fiber, 9 mg calcium.

Healthier Hummus

My original recipe called for ⅔ cup of olive oil and ½ cup of tahini. I reduced the fat considerably and used some of the chickpea liquid to provide moistness. As a shortcut, use canned chickpeas.

> 2 cups cooked chickpeas or 19 oz (540 ml) can chickpeas
> ¼ cup fresh parsley
> 3 cloves garlic (or see "Hummus with Roasted Garlic" under "Variations")
> 1 tbsp olive oil
> 2 tbsp tahini (sesame paste)
> 3 tbsp fresh lemon juice
> salt and pepper, to taste
> ½ tsp ground cumin
> dash of cayenne pepper or Tabasco sauce

1. Drain chickpeas, reserving about ½ cup of the liquid. (If using canned chickpeas, rinse under cold running water to remove excess sodium; drain well.)

2.   Process parsley and garlic until finely minced, about 15 seconds. Add chickpeas and process until puréed. Add remaining ingredients and process until very smooth, adding enough of reserved chickpea liquid for a creamy texture. Processing time will be about 3 minutes. Chill before serving. Serve as a dip with raw or steamed vegetables, crackers or toasted pita wedges. Great as a spread with raw veggies or low GI breads, crackers, or homemade carbs (above).

Yield: About 2 cups. Hummus keeps about 1 week in the refrigerator. Do not freeze.

23 calories per tbsp, 1.1 g fat (0.1 g saturated), 0 mg cholesterol, 1 g protein, 3 g carbohydrate, 1 mg sodium, 34 mg potassium, trace iron, <1 g fiber, 7 mg calcium.

Notes:

- *If desired, omit oil and increase tahini to 3 tablespoons. Although tahini is fairly high in fat, it contains important nutrients such as zinc, iron and calcium, and also provides flavor. Tahini can be found in supermarkets, Middle Eastern groceries or health food stores.*
- *To lower the fat in tahini, discard oil that comes to the top of the jar. Less fat, same flavor!*
- *For a handy light and nutritious meal, spread a pita with any of the variations of Healthier Hummus (see below). Top with sliced tomatoes and cucumber, red onion, red pepper (or roasted pepper strips) and sprouts. Great for the lunch box along with some fresh fruit and a thermos of soup!*

Variations:

- ***Skinnier Hummus:*** *Omit oil and tahini; add 1 green onion, minced. One serving contains 65 calories and 1 gram of fat.*
- ***Hummus with Roasted Garlic:*** *Use 1 head of roasted garlic in previous recipe.*

279

- **_Hummus with Roasted Red Peppers:_** _Add ½ cup roasted red peppers (homemade or from the jar) to chickpeas. Process until fine. Blend in remaining ingredients until smooth._
- **_White or Black Bean Spread:_** _Instead of chickpeas, substitute white kidney beans or black beans. Instead of the bean liquid, thin the mixture with a couple of spoonfuls of non-fat yogurt._

Mexican 7-Layer Dip

You'll love this de-liteful version of a formerly fat-laden dip. Did you know that avocado is a fruit? Buy two avocados when making this recipe. Mash one to use as a facial. Use the other one for this recipe. You'll look great and so will the dip!

119 oz can (540 ml) black beans
¾ cup fat-free or light mayonnaise
¾ cup low-fat sour cream
1 tsp chili powder
½ tsp each of cumin and dried oregano
6 green onions, chopped
½ cup sliced black olives
2 tomatoes, diced and drained
1 medium avocado, diced
1 tbsp fresh lemon juice
¾ cup grated low-fat cheddar cheese

1. Drain beans; rinse well. Mash beans and spread evenly in a 10-inch pie plate or quiche dish. In a small bowl, mix mayonnaise, yogurt cheese and spices. Spread over beans. Arrange green onions, olives and tomatoes in layers. Mix avocado with lemon juice and spread over tomatoes. Sprinkle with cheese. Cover tightly with plastic wrap and chill. Serve with Pita or Tortilla Chips (see page 272).

Yield: About 6 cups (18 to 24 servings). Do not freeze.

13 calories per tbsp, 0.5 g fat (0.2 g saturated), <1 mg cholesterol, <1 g protein, 2 g carbohydrate, 42 mg sodium, 19 mg potassium, trace iron, <1 g fiber, 13 mg calcium.

Ranch-Style Dressing (or Dip)
(See recipe, page 112.)

Red Lentil Paté
(See recipe, page 129.)

Spinach and Herb Dip
A favorite in my cooking classes!

2 cups non-fat natural yogurt
½ of a 10 oz (300 g) pkg frozen spinach, thawed and squeezed dry
2 cloves garlic, minced
4 green onions, minced
1 medium carrot, minced
¼ cup fresh parsley, minced
2 tbsp minced fresh dill (or 1 tsp dried)
1 tbsp minced fresh basil (or 1 tsp dried)
⅓ cup fat-free or light mayonnaise
salt and pepper, to taste
1 tsp lemon juice
1 round pumpernickel bread (optional)

1. Place yogurt in a strainer lined with a paper coffee filter or cheesecloth. Place over a bowl and let drain in the fridge for 2 to 3 hours. Combine drained yogurt with remaining ingredients and blend well. (If using a processor, first mince the veggies, then blend in remaining ingredients with quick on/off turns.) Chill dip before serving to blend flavors.

Yield: About 2½ cups of dip. Dip keeps for 3 or 4 days in the refrigerator.

9 calories per tbsp, 0 g fat (0 g saturated), trace cholesterol, <1 g protein, 2 g carbo-hydrate, 22 mg sodium, 38 mg potassium, trace iron, trace fiber, 19 mg calcium.

Notes:
- *No time to drain the yogurt? Use ¾ cup un-drained yogurt and increase mayonnaise to ¾ cup.*
- *Use a sharp knife to cut frozen package of spinach in half. Wrap and freeze the unused portion.*

Super Salsa (Uncooked)

This fresh salsa makes a delicious dip for crudités or Pita or Tortilla Chips (see page 272). It's also great with grilled fish, chicken or burgers.

4–5 large, ripe tomatoes (or 8 Italian plum tomatoes), finely chopped
2 cloves garlic, crushed
½ cup coriander/cilantro or parsley, minced
1 jalapeno pepper, seeded and minced
2 tbsp fresh basil, minced (or 1 tsp dried)
¼ cup green onions, chopped
2 tsp olive oil, to taste
2 tbsp fresh lemon juice, to taste
salt and pepper, to taste
dash of cayenne or Tabasco sauce
1 tbsp tomato paste, optional

1. Combine all ingredients except tomato paste and mix well. (The processor does a quick job of chopping the vegetables.) If mixture seems watery, add tomato paste. Season to taste.

Yield: About 3 cups. Serve with Pita or Tortilla Chips (see page 272). Salsa keeps for 2 to 3 days in the refrigerator in a tightly closed container. Do not freeze.

5 calories per tbsp, 0.2 g fat (0 g saturated), 0 mg cholesterol, trace protein, <1 g carbohydrate, 1 mg sodium, 32 mg potassium, trace iron, trace fiber, 2 mg calcium.

Notes:

- *Italian plum tomatoes make a thicker salsa than regular tomatoes because they're firmer, with less seeds and juice.*
- *Don't rub your eyes after handling hot peppers. It's a smart idea to wear rubber gloves. Don't forget to remove the gloves before touching your eyes … or you'll be yelling "eye, eye, eye!"*

Variations:

- ***Mediterranean Salsa:*** *Follow recipe for Super Salsa, but add 6 pitted and chopped black olives and 3 tablespoons drained capers. Use 1 tablespoon each of lemon juice and balsamic vinegar.*
- ***Black Bean Salsa:*** *Add a pinch of cumin and 1 cup of canned black beans, rinsed and drained, to Super Salsa.*
- ***Salsa Salad Dressing:*** *Combine leftover salsa with a little tomato juice or V8 vegetable cocktail in the food processor. Process with 6 or 8 on/off turns.*
- ***Speedy Salsa Gazpacho:*** *Combine ½ cup of chopped cucumber, ½ cup chopped green pepper, 1½ cups tomato juice and 2 cups of salsa. Add crushed garlic, salt and freshly ground pepper. Serve chilled.*
- ***Salsa Supper in a Snap:*** *Cut several large squares of cooking parchment or aluminum foil. Place a boneless chicken breast or fish fillet on each square. Top each one with a spoonful of salsa. Seal packets tightly. Arrange on a baking sheet and place in a preheated 400°F oven. Fish cooks in 10 to 12 minutes and chicken breasts take 20 to 25 minutes. Easy and good!*

Thousand Island Dressing (or Dip)

(See recipe, page 117.)

Tuna and Black Bean Antipasto

My sister (and best friend!) Rhonda Matias helped me create this delicious new way to prepare an old Winnipeg classic. The ingredient list is long, but it's quick to make. It's worth it!

1 medium onion
1 stalk celery
2 carrots
1 red pepper, cored and seeded
1 cup cauliflower florets
2-6½ oz (184 g) cans solid white tuna
10 oz (300 ml) can sliced mushrooms
½ cup sliced green stuffed olives
½ cup sliced black olives
1 cup sweet mixed pickles
19 oz can (540 ml) black beans
1½ cups ketchup
1½ cups bottled chili sauce
1 cup salsa (bottled or homemade)
½ tsp each of chili and garlic powder
¼ tsp each of rosemary and oregano
2 tbsp lemon juice
1 tbsp Worcestershire sauce
1 tsp sugar

1. Cut onion, celery, carrots and red pepper into ½-inch pieces. Break up cauliflower into bite-sized pieces. Blanch vegetables in boiling water for 1 to 2 minutes. They should still be somewhat crunchy. (Or sprinkle them with 2 tablespoons water and microwave covered on HIGH for 3 to 4 minutes.) Rinse under cold running water. Drain well. Drain tuna, mushrooms, olives, pickles and beans.

2. Combine all ingredients together in a large bowl and mix well. (Don't mash the tuna; it should be somewhat chunky in texture.) Adjust seasonings to taste. Serve chilled with crackers or in a mound on a bed of assorted salad greens.

Yield: About 12 cups. This keeps approximately 2 weeks in the refrigerator, or freezes beautifully.

12 calories per tbsp, 0.2 g fat (0 g saturated), <1 mg cholesterol, <1 g protein, 2 g carbohydrate, 96 mg sodium, 28 mg potassium, trace iron, trace fiber, 4 mg calcium.

Note:
- To reduce sodium, rinse black beans, olives and sweet mixed pickles under cold running water for at least 1 minute, then pat dry. You can also use low-sodium ketchup, make your own salsa and omit Worcestershire sauce.

■ OTHER STUFF

Homemade "Sun-Dried" Tomatoes

Sun-dried tomatoes are great for salads, dressings, sauces, casseroles, dips, pizza, pasta, rice and other grains. Nutrient values were not available for homemade sun-dried tomatoes, so my analysis is for store-bought. These are fabulous!

1 dozen (or more) ripe Italian plum tomatoes
salt, to taste

1. Preheat oven to 200°F. Rinse tomatoes. Either cut them in half or slice thinly. Pat dry with paper towels. Spread on foil-lined baking sheet(s) sprayed with non-stick spray. Sprinkle lightly with salt. Bake at 200°F until shrivelled, about 8 hours or overnight. Store in a tightly sealed container in the fridge. They'll keep several weeks. To rehydrate

tomatoes, cover with boiling water. Soak for 10 minutes. Drain well.

35 calories per ¼ cup, 0.4 g fat (0.1 g saturated), 0 mg cholesterol, 2 g protein, 8 g carbohydrate, 283 mg sodium, 463 mg potassium, 1 mg iron, 2 g fiber, 15 mg calcium.

Notes:

- *Small Italian plum tomatoes (Roma) are ideal because of their low juice content.*
- *Fat-saving secret: store-bought sun-dried tomatoes are often packed in oil. Rinse thoroughly with boiling water to remove the oil; pat dry. Oil left in the jar can be used for salad dressings, or instead of olive oil to sauté vegetables for pilafs and grain-based dishes.*

Pita Pizzas

(See recipe, page 173.) Also refer to "Well-Dressed Pitas," page 175.

Roasted Red Peppers

Roasted yellow and orange peppers also taste great. Very delicious, very versatile!

1. Preheat the broiler or grill. Broil or grill peppers until their skin is black-ened and blistered. Keep turning them until they're uniformly charred. Immediately put them into a brown paper bag or covered bowl and let cool. Scrape off the skin using a paring knife. Rinse quickly under cold water to remove any bits of charred skin. Pat dry. Cut in half and dis-card stem, core and seeds. If desired, cut peppers into strips. These freeze beautifully.

20 calories per pepper, 0.1 g fat (0 g saturated), 0 mg cholesterol, <1 g protein, 5 g carbohydrate, 2 mg sodium, 121 mg potassium, trace iron, 1 g fiber, 7 mg calcium.

Notes:

- *If you have a gas stove, roast one pepper at a time over a high flame using a long-handled fork. Buy peppers in the fall when prices are cheap. Broil or barbecue a large bunch of them at one time, then cool and peel.*

Discard the stem, core and seeds. Freeze in small containers.

- *An easy way to freeze these is to place roasted peppers halves or pieces in a single layer on a foil-lined baking sheet. When frozen, transfer them to freezer bags and store in the freezer until needed. Defrost as many as you need at one time.*
- *Roasted red pepper strips are absolutely wonderful in sandwiches. They're also yummy when mixed with Simply Basic Vinaigrette (page 115), bottled low-cal Italian dressing or balsamic vinegar.*
- *Pureéd roasted red peppers add a smoky taste to salad dressings, soups, sauces, dips and dressings.*

Smoked Salmon and Pumpernickel Hors D'Oeuvres

Perfect for lunch or a snack. An easy appetizer from student Gloria Schachter, a great proofreader and friend!

> 6 slices of square pumpernickel bread
> 5 tsp honey-style mustard
> ½ tsp each of Dijon and prepared mustard
> 6 oz smoked salmon (lox)
> fresh dill sprigs, to garnish

1. Spread each slice of bread with combined mustards. Cover with a layer of smoked salmon. Trim off crusts. Cut each slice into 4 squares or triangles. (Can be made several hours ahead, covered tightly and refrigerated until 10 to 15 minutes before serving time.) Garnish with dill.

Yield: 24 pieces. Can be frozen if very well wrapped.

28 calories per piece, 0.6 g fat (0.1 g saturated), 2 mg cholesterol, 2 g protein, 4 g carbohydrate, 116 mg sodium, 28 mg potassium, trace iron, trace fiber, 6 mg calcium.

Sun-Dried Tomato and Olive Pinwheels

Use dry pack sun-dried tomatoes, or make them yourself (see recipe, page 285).

1 cup light cream cheese
¼ cup sun-dried tomatoes
¼ cup green onions, minced
1 clove garlic, minced
2 tbsp pitted black olives, finely chopped
3 whole-wheat or flour tortillas (or very thin pitas, split in half crosswise)

1. Cover sun-dried tomatoes with boiling water and let stand for 10 minutes. Drain well; pat dry. Cut into small pieces with scissors or a sharp knife.
2. Place cheese in a bowl with remaining ingredients except tortillas; mix lightly to blend. (Do not use a processor or the mixture will become too thin.) Spread in a thin layer on tortillas. (Leave a ½-inch border around the bottom edge of each tortilla so that cheese will not ooze out when rolled up.)
3. Roll up tightly, cover and refrigerate until needed. (These can be eaten like a roll-up, if you wish.) When needed, trim off ends. (They're for nibbling!) Slice each roll on a slight angle into 8 slices. Arrange on a large platter lined with lettuce or spinach leaves. Serve chilled.

Yield: About 24 pinwheels or 3 roll-ups.

19 calories per pinwheel, 0.2 g fat (0 g saturated), trace cholesterol, 1 g protein, 4 g carbohydrate, 47 mg sodium, 57 mg potassium, trace iron, <1 g fiber, 22 mg calcium.

■ SWEET STUFF

The following make the perfect snacks when you crave something sweet and not savory!

Carrot Muffins
(See recipe, page 73.)

Chocolate and Mint Leaves
(See recipe, page 250.)

Chocolate Chip Bran-ana Muffins
(See recipe, page 250.)

Chunky Monkey
(See recipe, page 253.)

Fruit Smoothies
(See recipe, page 51.)

Homemade Applesauce
(See recipe, page 52.)

Hot Chocolate (Cocoa)
(See recipe, page 252.)

Mary's Best Bran-ana Bread
(See recipe, page 73.)

Mock Banana Soft Ice Cream
(See recipe, page 254.)

Orange Creamy Dream
(See recipe, page 255.)

Rozie's Magical Carrot Muffins
(See recipe, page 75.)

Strawberry and Banana Frozen Yogurt
(See recipe, page 56.)

Strawberry Buttermilk Sherbet
(See recipe, page 255.)

GLYCEMIC INDEX TABLES

LOW GLYCEMIC INDEX FOODS (55 OR LESS)

Note: The following foods are listed alphabetically. Their corresponding GI values are based on a standard "single" serving.

All Bran	42
Apple juice, unsweetened	40
Apple	38
Baked beans in tomato sauce	48
Banana	55
Butter beans	31
Carrots, boiled	49
Cherries	22
Chickpeas, canned	42
Dried apricots	31
Fettucine pasta, cooked al dente	32
Grapefruit	25
Green grapes	46
Kiwi fruit	52
Lentil soup	44
Low-fat fruit yogurt	33
Low-fat yogurt with low GI sweetener	14
Macaroni	45
Milk chocolate	49
Noodles	40
Oatmeal made with water	42
Orange juice	46
Orange	44

LOW GLYCEMIC INDEX FOODS (55 OR LESS)	
Note: The following foods are listed alphabetically. Their corresponding GI values are based on a standard "single" serving.	
Peach	42
Pearl barley	25
Pear	38
Peas	48
Potato chips	54
Raw oat bran	55
Red lentil	26
Roasted and salted peanuts	14
Skimmed milk	32
Special K	54
Stone ground wholegrain bread	53
Sweet corn	55
Tomato soup, canned	38
White spaghetti, cooked al dente	41
Whole milk	27
Wholegrain spaghetti, cooked al dente	37

Source: Weight Loss Resources Ltd., 2007.

MEDIUM/MODERATE GLYCEMIC INDEX FOODS (56 TO 69)

Note: The following foods are listed alphabetically. Their corresponding GI values are based on a standard "single" serving.

Apricots, canned in syrup	64
Basmati rice	58
Boiled potatoes	56
Cantaloupe melon	67
Cheese and tomato pizza	60
Coca cola	63
Couscous	65
Croissant	67
Crumpet, toasted	69
Digestive biscuit	59
Honey	58
Ice cream	61
Mars bar	68
Muesli, non-toasted	56
New potatoes	62
Pineapple, fresh	66
Pita bread	57
Raisins	64
Rye bread	65
Shortbread biscuit	64
Shredded Wheat	67
Sultanas	56
Wholegrain bread	69

Source: Weight Loss Resources Ltd., 2007.

HIGH GLYCEMIC INDEX FOODS (70 OR MORE)

Note: The following foods are listed alphabetically. Their corresponding GI values are based on a standard "single" serving.

Bagel	72
Baguette	95
Bran flakes	74
Cheerios	74
Cornflakes	84
French fries	75
Jacket potato	85
Jelly beans	80
Mashed potato	70
Parsnips, boiled	97
Puffed wheat	89
Rice cakes	82
Rice Krispies	82
Watermelon	72
White bread	70
White rice, steamed	98

Source: Weight Loss Resources Ltd., 2007.

BEST LOW GI CHOICES AT A GLANCE

Note: All of the following foods are good low GI choices. However, within each category they are listed in order of best to worst.

Beverages
Soymilk
Apple juice (unsweetened)

Breads
100% stone-ground
Whole wheat or multigrain
Made with wholegrain flour
Cracked or sprouted
Whole wheat
Dark, heavy, coarse breads with intact whole grains, seeds, nuts, flax seeds, oats, or oat bran
Pumpernickel
Rye
Sourdough
Whole-wheat pita bread
Whole-wheat tortilla

Cereals
All-Bran®
Bran Buds®
Fiber One®
Muesli
Rolled Oats (old-fashioned oatmeal)
Corn flakes/Chex®/Pops®
Puffed wheat or rice
Rice Krispies®/Chex

Dairy Products
All milk
Cooked pudding and custard
"Light" (artificially or fructose-sweetened) or plain yogurt
Ice cream

Fruits
Apples
Apricots
Berries
Cherries
Citrus fruits
Grapes
Nectarines
Peaches
Pears
Plums
Prunes
Strawberries
Juices

Juices
Unsweetened juice—apple, grapefruit, orange, tomato

Legumes and Beans
Baked beans
Black beans
Black-eyed peas
Butter beans
Cannellini beans
Chickpeas
Kidney beans

Lentils
Mung beans
Pinto beans
Soy beans
Split peas

Pasta and Grains
Arborio rice
Barley
Basmati rice
Brown rice
Buckwheat
Bulgur
Corn
Glutinous rice (sticky Chinese rice)
Jasmine rice
Pasta cooked al dente
Tortellini
Uncle Ben's® Converted® Long-Grain Rice (not instant)
Wild rice

Vegetables
All green leafy vegetables
All "non-starchy" vegetables (except beets)
Carrots
Corn
New potatoes
Peas
Sweet potatoes
Yams
Sweetened vegetable juices and juice drinks
Fava beans

Baked and mashed potatoes
Beets
Parsnips
Pumpkin
Rutabaga

Source: Compiled using the GI database on www.glycemicindex.com, *2006.*

RECIPE INDEX

A

B

D

E

F

G

2619510R00168

Made in the USA
San Bernardino, CA
13 May 2013